Psychiatry for Students
Fifth Edition

Psychiatry for Students

Fifth Edition

DAVID STAFFORD-CLARK
M.D., F.R.C.P., F.R.C.Psych., D.P.M.

Consultant Emeritus to Guy's Hospital and Medical School in the Department of Psychiatry; lately Consultant to the Institute of Psychiatry of the University of London, and to the Bethlem Royal and Maudsley Hospitals

and

ANDREW C. SMITH
M.B., B.Chir., M.R.C.P. Edin., M.R.C.Psych., D.P.M.

Hon. Lecturer and Hon. Consultant in the Department of Psychiatry, Guy's Hospital Medical School; Consultant Psychiatrist at Bexley Hospital, Greenwich District Hospital and Dreadnought Seamen's Hospital.

London
GEORGE ALLEN & UNWIN
Boston   Sydney

First Published 1964
Second Edition 1966
Third Edition 1967
Fourth Edition 1974
Fifth Edition 1978
Reprinted 1979 (with corrections)
Third impression 1981

GEORGE ALLEN & UNWIN LTD
40 Museum Street, London WC1A 1LU

© George Allen & Unwin (Publishers) Ltd, 1964, 1966, 1967, 1974, 1978.

New material in this Fifth Edition
© David Stafford-Clark and Andrew C. Smith, 1978, 1979

ISBN 0 04 132016 6 Hardback
0 04 132017 4 Paperback

British Library Cataloguing in Publication Data

Stafford-Clark, David
  Psychiatry for students. – 5th ed.
  1. Psychiatry
  I. Title   II. Smith, Andrew C
  616.8′9′   RC454   77–30586

  ISBN 0–04–132016–6
  ISBN 0–04–132017–4   Pbk

Printed in Great Britain
in 10 on 12 point Times Roman
by Billing & Sons Limited, Guildford, London and Worcester

Foreword

Even a textbook must have a philosophy. For whatever the information it seeks to impart, whatever the facts it attempts to describe, it will also contain, and explicitly or implicitly will convey, a point of view. There are already a number of textbooks about psychiatry in existence; the point of view from which this one is written is that clinical study of the subject must include an appreciation of how it feels to be the patient.

Never to forget this aspect when actually confronted by someone distressed in mind or body, is to retain a key to understanding, to a detached but sincere compassion, and to an objective wisdom based upon the interpretation of experience. This will always remain the foundation of clinical medicine, whose ultimate function and essential justification is simply the relief of human suffering.

Preface to the Fifth Edition

The preface to the 4th Edition in 1974 contained two predictions: the first implicit, the second explicit. The first has fortunately been vindicated by time and the generous energy of Dr Andrew Smith, now an established Consultant in the N.H.S. and a member of the Academic Department of Psychiatry of Guy's Hospital Medical School. He was once the 'thoughtful chief assistant' who gave me such characteristically sound and categorical advice about the life-span of a textbook. He has now accepted the responsibility of its revision, updating and future. Everything new in this edition is his. It is a singularly gratifying conclusion to my own endeavours in this respect.

The second prediction (that the 4th Edition would comprise two separate but related volumes, the Second being an original exposition of Child and Adolescent Psychiatry by my friend and colleague Dr G. F. Vaughan) has unfortunately not materialised. Instead we revert to the original single volume, with a new section on Child Psychiatry by Dr Smith. It is my belief, as well as my hope, that this 5th edition will live up to the reputation accorded to its predecessors.

'Psychiatry for Students' declared its credentials, and acknowledged its philosophy in the original foreword to the first edition. In entrusting this and future editions to the sole responsibility of Andrew Smith, I acknowledge unreservedly that for this particular task he was my first and only choice; and I am truly delighted that he has accepted the challenge with that meticulous diligence and honest independent intelligence which has commanded my respect since we first worked together. Let the outcome speak for itself: eclectic clinical psychiatry is here to stay.

DAVID STAFFORD-CLARK

It only remains for me to express my thanks, especially to David Stafford-Clark for his absolutely unstinting loyalty and support. I profited from suggestions made by Professor Michael Gelder of Oxford and Professor F. A. Jenner of Sheffield, and I am grateful to them.

D. H. C. Smith and A. P. C. Smith helped me with the diagram and the index.

I am profoundly grateful to my secretary, Mrs. F. Downing, for typing the manuscript and remaining such a very good friend.

A.C.S.

Preface to the First Edition

The preface to a new textbook may be offered in excuse for having
written it, in explanation of its aims, or in acknowledgement of sources
of help or inspiration.

The book begins with a foreword, and no further excuse will be made.
Its aim is to inform; if possible with interest: and the student to whom
it is addressed may be medical, dental, sociological, psychological or
philosophical; undergraduate or postgraduate; or perhaps simply
interested.

Acknowledgements could be legion – and perhaps they should: but
the more numerous they become the less adequate would they be. So
may I simply record that I owe more than I can say to my former
teachers and patients for their example and endurance, to my students
for whatever they have taught me about teaching, and to my family and
friends for their affection and encouragement.

Miss D. M. Harlow typed and retyped the recurring manuscripts,
successive registrars and housemen kept me and the proofs in order,
and my secretary Miss Rosbrook maintained the fabric of my professional life, while my wife continued to sustain everything else about me
during the writing of the book. The value of the invited contributions
of Dr G. F. Vaughan and Lady Williams is self-evident; and equally
valuable was the help I received from Dr A. K. M. Macrae in elucidating
for me the differences between English and Scottish Law for the
appendix to Chapter 15: I can only repeat my personal thanks to each,
for their contributions.

Throughout all, the publishers have remained my friends.

D.S.-C.

Preface to Second Edition

A call for a second edition within a year of the publication of the first is a tangible compliment: and gives me the opportunity of heeding some of my more constructive critics. The section on the detailed technique of hypnosis, together with Appendix II, has been omitted. The first edition provided them with original publication, but it would have been redundant to have retained them. In their place room has been made for additional material on chronic schizophrenia, a more specific reference to the psychiatric aspects of epilepsy, and a note on the application of learning theory to the treatment of neuroses. Aversion treatment has been left to those who favour it.

Two other general matters perhaps require brief comment. Recently published studies by my eminent friend and senior colleague. Dr Eliot Slater, have seemed to some postgraduate students to imply that the concepts of hysterical personality and hysterical symptoms must now be regarded with suspicion. My own reading of his work is rather that, while the concept of hysterical personality lacks a genetic foundation, the diagnosis of hysterical symptoms is an indication for accurate judgement and careful clinical assessment of the entire predicament of the patient: but not that hysteria is an outmoded concept, nor that its recognition is unimportant, still less to be avoided on principle. Neither of the relevant sections have therefore been amended; and indeed I venture to hope that attention to the principles enunciated in the first part of Chapter 7 will protect readers against those very misconceptions with which Dr Eliot Slater has been rightly concerned.

The second point concerns dementia. Professor Erwin Stengel, an acknowledged expert on classification, whom I also hold in high regard, has taken me to task for my use of the terms primary and secondary in this connection, to denote respectively idiopathic and symptomatic manifestations of brain disease. I take his point, particularly as primary dementia is used in an entirely different sense in the World Health Organization International Classification of Diseases: Section V: Mental, Psychoneurotic, and Personality Disorders; where dementia is widely included under Schizophrenic disorders (300, 0–7) as well as in the general group of Senile, Pre-senile, and other degenerative psychoses (304–309): whereas in the Standard Classification of the American Psychiatric Association the term dementia is not used at all.

But after careful reflection I have remained unrepentant. My own definitions and classification are logical and pragmatic; and as used in this book will enable the student to sort as well as comprehend his clinical experience, before resorting either to the International Classification or the American Psychiatric Association, whose aims are not primarily clinical at all. Moreover the use of the term dementia in the context of schizophrenia, in the International Classification of the World Health Organization, seems to me simply to prolong an obsolete terminological confusion which is already over fifty years out of date.

Consideration of these matters has produced a preface to the second edition considerably longer than the preface to the first. But the text book itself remains unswollen.

D.S.-C.

Preface to the Fourth Edition

One of my most thoughtful chief assistants, talking about textbooks in general, once said to me that he thought the useful life of a textbook was, at most, fifteen years.

After that, he said, it might be preserved in archives as a historical document – if it had been good enough – but to continue publishing it to keep it in circulation ultimately succeeded only in murdering its original image and impact. Better to hand over the textbook chore to someone else. Someone younger, he added, with a reputation still to make, and a new title; not tied to an established but ageing tradition.

I believe him. This therefore will be the last time I shall up-date this book, which has been so generously received by my colleagues and students all over the world, since it first appeared in hardback in 1964. Perhaps my adviser or one of his contemporaries will help the publishers to keep the book alive for its next five years – but as a start we have revised it very dramatically. It will now come in two volumes, each no larger than the original, and available either as a package or separately.

Volume I, by me, has a new appendix on Clinical Psychology by Dr Donald Bannister, replacing Mrs Jessie Williams's graceful original contribution. I am particularly indebted to Dr George Hsu for suggesting most of the updating material included.

Volume II will be by Dr Gerard Vaughan, who will devote it entirely to Child and Adolescent Psychiatry, and will cover the latest developments in the psychology of emotional maturation, and the emergence of the personality. The original chapter on this subject will therefore be omitted from my volume, with everything else that will be covered in Volume II. Volume I will deal essentially and exclusively with adults no longer answerable to parental *angst*.

We all hope this will improve the contribution and make the total field complementary and comprehensive. But as always, the reader must be the final judge.

D.S.-C.

Contents

behaviour therapy – hypnosis – abreaction, using physical
methods – planning treatment – conclusions – references and
further reading.

Chapter 1

The Nature of the Subject

Definition and Preliminary Considerations

Psychiatry is that part of medicine which is primarily concerned with disorders of thought, feeling, and behaviour. In one sense all illness or injury, and indeed all suffering of any kind, involves disorder of feeling; and this is one of the reasons why the basic principles of psychiatry are vital to a proper understanding of medicine and surgery as a whole. But the special province of psychiatry is the understanding of those disorders of subjective experience or objective behaviour which are themselves a cause of disability.

They may be primary, or secondary to some other illness or structural damage. The disturbance of experience or behaviour to which they give rise may be apparent to the sufferer, in which case he is said to have insight into the nature of his illness; or he may be entirely unaware that he is ill or disabled in this way, and may attribute his experience or predicament to changes in the world around him. All this every doctor must be able to acknowledge, to understand, to diagnose, and at least in some degree to treat. Psychiatry in fact includes in its concern that most human aspect of human beings, their awareness of themselves, and their capacity to communicate with each other.

Understood in this sense the field is a wide one: it includes the normal emotional reaction to sickness or physical disaster of any kind, as well as the effects of emotion upon bodily function and structure; particularly the abnormal effects of excessive and undischarged emotion.

Disorders arising out of such repercussion of emotion upon bodily function or structure are often called psychosomatic illnesses; but although their particular study has proved one of the most rewarding and illuminating aspects of modern psychological medicine, their greatest importance lies in the light they have cast upon the aetiology of illness in general. It is in the psychosomatic approach to many of the problems of general medicine, surgery, and obstetrics, as well as in the field of paediatrics, that psychiatry has made one of its greatest contributions to clinical knowledge and understanding.

Also included within the field of psychiatry are those disorders arising from a failure of function of the brain and nervous system, whether due to imperfect development, to diseases, or to injury. Finally there are those illnesses which present as abnormalities of behaviour, adjustment, or adaptation of human mental life in response to environment; such abnormality being related to hereditary or constitutional factors, to the impact of excessive stress, or to causes as yet incompletely known.

This latter group of illnesses are sometimes collectively called *functional* mental disorders; they are of various kinds and have been variously classified. A distinction is frequently made in practice between one group of mental disorders which are called neuroses, and another which are called psychoses. Whether its fundamental validity is accepted or not, few will deny that in practice this distinction is useful and convenient. Under its terms, neuroses are those disorders of emotional and intellectual functioning which do not deprive a patient of contact with reality; while the psychoses are characterized by a profound and essential disturbance in the patient's appreciation of the nature of his environment and his response to it.

The practical implications of this distinction can be illustrated by an example of one of the simplest sources of distress from which a patient may suffer; the fear of illness. If a patient presents with palpitations, and a sense of constriction in his chest, and eventually and somewhat ashamedly confesses that he is afraid that his heart may cease to beat or that he is liable to drop dead after exertion, this may well prove to be a symptom of anxiety which can reasonably be regarded as neurotic. But if his elaboration of the complaint reveals that he believes that his heart has stopped already, in response to atomic fall-out directed specifically against him, and that he is now living on borrowed time, these bizarre and delusional ideas suggest that the underlying disorder is psychotic. While this is enough to exemplify the meaning of the distinction, its signficance in terms of the nature and severity of any illness to which it is applied will be developed in later stages of this book.

Enough has been said to show that all these afflictions will tend in varying degree to produce an extremely disagreeable effect upon the patient who suffers from them; primarily an impairment of his capacity both to interpret his own experiences, and to communicate them to others; and secondarily, and arising from this, an impairment in his capacity to achieve a normal relationship with other people. Indeed, it is a sad but constant experience that patients attempting to explain their feelings and troubles, when these are related to disturbances of their mental life, nearly always meet with hostility, contempt, or disbelief on the part of those to whom they entrust their confidence.

Any practising doctor is bound to encounter disorders of this kind in his patients, and must be prepared to listen without ridicule or contempt to the patient's own account of what seems to be happening to him, and the way in which he is experiencing it. Nothing is gained by dismissing such testimony as absurd or unreasonable; because either the patient knows this already and is very unhappy about it, or he does not know it, and is therefore bound to resent so insensitive and palpably obtuse an attitude, since it shows him that the doctor does not even understand what he is trying to say.

Normally it does not require a great deal of effort or imagination to put oneself in the patient's place, when his complaint is largely physical. Patients with structural illness or injury, in this respect at least, are in a relatively fortunate category; for even though their description of their sufferings may be clinically inaccurate, it is usually recognized and accepted by doctors without difficulty. Sensing this, some patients suffering from symptoms of fear, unhappiness, or emotional tension, will seek to convey them in physical terms, to gain at least the immediate sympathy and help of the person to whom they are turning. Against the neurotic patient, with his apparently indefatigable capacity for continued complaint, seemingly unrelated to any objective pathology, many a harassed physician has felt driven to attack as the best method of defence. The patient's reaction to this is often to cling yet more stubbornly to the idea of a physical basis for his symptoms, and to describe them in physical terms. Not only does this seem more respectable to him; he assumes that it will also seem more respectable to his doctor. Moreover, many patients' powers of description, introspection, and self-analysis are sufficiently limited to make physical complaint the only way in which they can experience or express their need of help.

The greater the element of emotional disturbance, whether the underlying disorder be structural or functional, the greater will be the discrepancy between the patient's understanding of what is happening, and his capacity to explain this to others, or to maintain a normal relationship with them in other ways. When the main source of a patient's distress is a disturbance of mood, intellect, or behaviour, of the kind which characterizes so many mental illnesses, this factor of the patient's own incapacity to understand what is happening, and the difficulty which other people may at first experience in accepting such a patient at all, may be crucial; and the task of understanding and treating patients suffering in this way will be correspondingly difficult. This is because our basic confidence in our capacity to understand our own feelings and those of other people, is an aspect of our lives which we normally take very much for granted: and we are therefore intrinsically handicapped in recognizing that a disruption of these capacities in mental illness is as much of an objective disability, and as little of a deliberate breach of the rules of good manners, taste, or behaviour, as is the display of physical symptoms or signs on the part of patients whose plight is immediately recognized as due to a failure of bodily structure or function. *There is in fact a wide gulf between the instinctive approach of the normal person to mental disaster on the one hand, and to physical on the other.* When in the past medicine has recognized the essential need to bridge this gulf, patients have been helped, and progress has been made. But when the gulf has yawned wide, the aims of medicine have been lost, and its principles have been betrayed.

Emotional Repercussions

Emotional disturbance in human beings tends to be in itself disturbing and even distasteful to others. Their instinctive reaction is at first surprise, then rejection, and finally outright hostility. Two lessons emerge from the study of man's reaction to those of his fellows who are mentally ill.

The first is that the general reaction of human beings to the difference or dangers, the illnesses or afflictions of other individuals, may sometimes be far less than the best of which they are capable, and lamentably remote from the ideals which they might profess and the principles to which they might subscribe. The second is that nevertheless man is not bound inevitably to betray himself, and that ideals and principles can be preserved in his attitude, if he will pay more particular attention to the plight of the individual who confronts him.

This has been fascinatingly underlined by the observations and subsequent speculations of a great naturalist, Professor Tinbergen, now at the University of Oxford, and formerly a professor of Zoology at the University of Leiden. During the process of attaching coloured leg rings to individual herring gulls so that he could identify them on future occasions in the course of observing the whole colony, he was struck by the behaviour of the rest of the colony towards a temporarily netted gull, furiously struggling in a hitherto unfamiliar and potentially dangerous predicament. At first they uttered loud cries of a kind usually associated with a warning to the whole flock; then they took off and flew away from this bird, circling round and watching him from a distance. Then some of them swooped in and made attacks on him as he continued to struggle helplessly. Normally this whole process was over in a few seconds, and the bird, with the harmless ring on his leg, was released. But the three stages of surprise and alarm, of withdrawal from his company, and finally of outright attack on him, were clearly seen in the reaction of his companions.

Tinbergen comments, 'One is tempted to compare this with human behaviour. In human society, primitive as well as civilized, a similar instinctive reaction is very strongly developed'. He goes on to stress 'the grave importance for human sociology to recognize the instinctive basis of such reactions, and to study them comparatively in other social species. . . .'.

Some alternative to this pattern of behaviour, whether it be mainly innate and instinctive or largely conditioned by society in its powerful pressure against deviant behaviour, by which we first deride, then reject, finally perhaps even attack the individual whose behaviour we do not or cannot accept, is of course indispensable if we are to raise ourselves above the level of animals in the way in which ultimately we treat each other. The doctor's example in handling his patients here must be impeccable. Sometimes this will not be easy. From what we have already learned of the impact of emotional disturbance upon communication between human beings, it begins to be clear that the key to a proper approach to such disturbance *whether or not* it occurs against a background of mental illness, is to attempt to understand the way in which this disturbance or illness is affecting the patient's relationship with others, and his power to interpret and communicate his own experiences. The frequently disruptive impact of such illness upon these two aspects of human existence, normally taken completely for granted, helps to explain why, throughout the history of mental illness, the attitude of the average person towards this type of catastrophe has been more often one of resentment or blame or fear, than of compassion, or a willingness to accept and understand.

Historical Consequences

The scope of this book does not include a detailed consideration of the history of psychiatry. Sources from which this may be sought are given in a brief bibliography at the end of this chapter.

Taken all in all, it amounts to a savage and sickening story. The concept of man as a whole being of infinite worth and potential dignity, originated in 400 BC by Hippocrates as a proper approach to the study of medicine, did not long survive him. Hippocrates had taught simply and consistently that the physician's task was to study the diseased individual, rather than disease as an abstract entity: the whole, and not the part. When his disciples forgot and betrayed these teachings they reopened the way to a cleavage which once again developed between mental illness and all other kinds of affliction; and once mental illness could be regarded as a thing apart, the fear and hostility latent in the attitude of men towards those whose behaviour they could not understand, largely determined the treatment accorded them.

Up to the beginning of the last century, patients suffering from mental illness were in general still so brutally treated that few of them had any chance of recovery. Their illness was maintained and indeed increased by isolation, darkness, cold, filth, starvation, purging, beating, and chains. It may now seem beyond belief that doctors and the public could contemplate other human beings naked, shivering, crusted with their own excrement, chained and starving in the dark on stone floors, without pity and without remorse. But they could, and they did, and it was only by the exertions and examples of exceptional men and women that our own standards have been raised above this appalling state.

A vivid example of the complacency with which Elizabethan

society accepted this state of affairs is given by a gay aside from Rosalind flirting with Orlando, in *As You Like It*:

'. . . Love is merely a madness. And I tell you *deserves as well* a whip and a dark cell as madmen do.'

The italics are ours: but there is nothing to suggest that Shakespeare was here concerned with irony or social criticism. This was simply a lighthearted maiden's coyness, whose underlying assumptions were shared unquestioningly by the audience.

When, some 200 years later, in 1793, Philippe Pinel, Physician Superintendent of the Bicêtre Hospital in Paris, removed the chains from patients under his care, he released by this act not simply the bodies of the patients, but ultimately the minds of his colleagues, from preoccupation with cruelty and fear as permissible ways of treating the mentally ill. Even today this shadow still lingers over the public attitude to treatment. Nothing but understanding, compassion and respect for the individual man or woman who is the patient, will ever finally dispel it.

Social Implications

Psychiatric disorder in its widest sense is one of the commonest and most important aspects of medicine as a whole. At a conservative estimate about a third of the complaints which bring patients to their general practitioner, have a significant psychogenic component. Of the patients referred for consultation at hospital out-patient departments, the percentage is probably higher still. The problem of relatively serious mental illness in the community as a whole, although beginning to yield to recent advances in treatment and understanding, is still colossal. The population of England is approximately 46 million people, the number of patients at present in mental hospitals is a little under 90,000. In addition there are just over 50,000 patients in mental handicap hospitals, and many more in other institutions and homes for the care and training of backward children and adults.

But actually the mental hospitals are still over-crowded. Moreover it has been reliably estimated that present facilities for residential training of mentally backward people are *less than half* the minimum required to give everyone in this position a chance to realize their ultimate potential, and to live and work productively in reasonable happiness in the community.

Nor are the social implications of psychiatric disorder confined to the personal distress which it may cause the sufferer or his family, or to the pressure on medical time and hospital beds. Carefully assessed research has shown that between one-quarter and one-third of all absence from work due to sickness is due to illnesses having an essentially emotional basis. Absenteeism through this cause is many times greater than that due to labour disputes.

In practice, what links psychiatry inescapably with general medicine, surgery, and obstetrics is the ultimate impossibility of treating states of mind apart from states of body, or states of body apart from states of mind. Had psychiatry made no greater contribution to the balance and equilibrium of the general medical curriculum than to endorse and emphasize this single fact, its contribution would still have been invaluable; for it has too often been the assumption in the past that, while bodily states had to be exhaustively observed and meticulously studied, mental states could either be taken for granted or dismissed as irrelevant, in the training and clinical approach of the doctor.

Where the clinical material of psychiatry tends to differ from that of the rest of medicine and surgery, however, is in the frequency with which the actual basis of communication between doctor and patient is involved in, and impaired by, the illness from which the patient is suffering. *The essential raw material of clinical psychiatry is therefore carefully observed behaviour*: the term behaviour being used here in its widest sense, to include speech and writing as well as action; what the patient says, as well as what he does. The precise nature of a patient's complaint may be of decisive diagnostic significance, in the absence of objective physical signs; while *clear-cut syndromes, capable of correct and verifiable diagnosis, may yet be found to rest upon no objectively demonstrable structural pathology of any kind*.

All this makes clinical psychiatry a difficult but never a dull subject. Dealing with so much that is inevitably intangible, it cannot afford to be vague or nebulous, woolly or imprecise. The degree of its proper understanding is a measure of a doctor, and distinguishes the true physician from the hack.

To thread his way through this tangled morass of apprehension, prejudice and misunderstanding, with accuracy, wisdom and compassion, to the prestige of his profession and the ultimate benefit of his patients, the doctor needs a clinical competence and a sound but imaginative technique in examination. These must be the foundation of his clinical approach.

References and Further Reading on History

The standard short textbook is *A short history of psychiatry* by E. H. Ackerknecht 1969, New York: Hafner; and the long one *A history of medical psychology* by G. Zilboorg 1941, New York: Norton.

In Britain, see *Mental disorder in earlier Britain* by Basil Clarke 1975, Cardiff, Univ. of Wales, for mediaeval period; *Three hundred years of psychiatry, 1535–1860*, R. Hunter and I. Macalpine's masterpiece, Oxford University Press, 1963; and *The historical development of British psychiatry, Volume 1*, by D. Leigh 1961: Pergamon, for especially the eighteenth and early nineteenth centuries.

Also *A history of the mental health services* by K. Jones 1972, London: Routledge and Kegan Paul, which gives full coverage of its subject from 1744 to 1971.

In *Psychiatry today* 1952: Pelican, the senior of the present authors writes fifty pages on the history of psychiatry.

Chapter 2

The Clinical Approach

The Presenting Complaint

As in general medicine and surgery, this consists in the discovery of the presenting complaint – or reason for the consultation, if the patient is not personally complaining of anything – followed by history and examination.

The first necessity is to permit the patient to tell his troubles in his own words. Particular attention should be paid to the very opening sentence, which may contain nuances which encapsulate in a subtle way the complexity of the situation. There is a world of difference between 'I'm a bit tense'; 'It's this terrible tension'; 'My doctor said I'm tense and sent me to you'; and 'I'm tense and my wife thought I should see a doctor'.

Then a few minutes' patient listening will often elicit a tale of woe whose degree of involvement of thought, feeling, and general experience may point clearly to the nature of the underlying diagnosis. A difficult decision for the doctor then follows: he has to choose how much of the interview to devote to listening to and recording the story as it unfolds in the patient's own way, and when to interrupt this by the need to collect information systematically under headings and ask the patient questions. There is no rule for this, because the different style of different patients interplays with the judgment of the doctor: sometimes the patient's account, scarcely prompted, furnishes nearly all the facts; on other occasions early intervention is essential to divert a circumstantial account which in itself will never provide enough information about the full background.

The next step is an adequate history whose foundation rests upon the following aetiological considerations:

(1) Heredity and constitution.
(2) Environmental factors; including past physiological, psychological, and social stresses, and present life situation.
(3) The cumulative effect of these two in producing disturbance of normal psychophysiological equilibrium.

FAMILY HISTORY

Family history is important for the light it throws upon the start which the patient had in life, as well as the stock from which he sprang. It should extend as far back as the grandparents on both sides of the family, and should include available information about first cousins, uncles and aunts, as well as parents, siblings and children. Specific inquiries should be made about the incidence of serious illness or 'nervous breakdown' in the family, and a picture obtained of the personalities of key relatives and of the family's way of life, traditions, hopes and disappointments. More intensive investigation may be undertaken in this field if there is evidence of a strong genetic factor in the illness.

In general, constitutional factors are of greatest importance in mental handicap, certain disturbances of drive and profound instability of mood, and schizophrenia; they are much less important in acute emotional reactions to severe environmental stress, and acquired patterns of behaviour arising from them.

PERSONAL HISTORY

Personal history carries the story from infancy up to the present personal, marital or occupational difficulties, tracing these and the development of personality which preceded them, through childhood and relationships with parents and siblings, schooldays and relationships with fellow-pupils and teachers, adolescence, with awakening of psychosexual needs and relationships with members of the same and opposite sex, adult life and the achievement of present relationships with fellow human beings and the rest of the world. Against the background of this life-story must be sought the readjustments, ambitions, day-dreams, and disappointments, which have contributed to shaping the character and behaviour of the patient.

HISTORY OF PREVIOUS ILLNESSES

This must cover all serious illnesses to which the patient has been subject, both structural and functional. Particular attention should be paid to unexplained absence from school or work, or vague periods of ill-health. It is always worthwhile inquiring whether the patient has ever had any kind of nervous breakdown, or suffered from a similar illness to the one which afflicts him now. If so, *patterns* should be sought, for example, was the precipitating event in each case a form of increased responsibility at work, or the need to suppress resentment at a feeling of unjust treatment by father, boss or Government. Alternatively, was there on each occasion a history of recurrent physical illness, or of neglecting prescribed medication, or every time a complex mixture of overwhelming stresses?

PERSONALITY BEFORE ILLNESS

This should be an assessment of the kind of person the patient was, in the estimation of a reliable relative, friend or other informant.

Examples: ? Energetic, bright, cheerful. . . .
           ? Always a worrier. . . .
           ? Bold or timid; boisterous or quiet kind of person.
           ? Conscientious or lackadaisical. . . .

The general level of mood, and capacity for relationship with other people, should be included, and on occasion a full and many-sided understanding of the make-up of the personality may be the main heading in comprehending the patient's problem.

HISTORY OF PRESENT COMPLAINT

Establish when the patient was last quite well. Establish the circumstances of onset of the condition and the symptoms at that time. Try to find out as much detail as possible about the situation in which the patient was placed when the illness began; his home environment, social situation, conditions at work, etc. Then trace the development of the illness from this onwards, noting the factors which influenced its course.

A complete history along these lines may take between half and three-quarters of an hour. The time will be well spent. Such a history will achieve two invaluable goals; not only will a complete picture of the patient as well as his complaint steadily emerge, but the rapport, gratitude and confidence felt by a patient for the doctor who thus displays so careful and penetrating an interest in his case, will itself prove of therapeutic importance.

PHYSICAL EXAMINATION

This is important whether or not there is any evidence of structural abnormality, and whether or not the patient complains of physical symptoms. Physical examination, gently but purposively and professionally undertaken, creates a bond of sympathy and acceptance. Anything the doctor may subsequently have to say to the patient will have gained strength and authority from this essential preliminary, even when physical findings indicative of structural disease have been neither anticipated nor obtained.

EXAMINATION OF MENTAL STATE

This is as definite and invaluable a technique as the physical examination, and is as indispensable a part of the equipment of the clinician. Observations should be assessed and recorded under the following headings:

(1) General appearance and behaviour
(2) Talk: manner and content
(3) Subjective state: mood and attitude to consultation
(4) Content of thought
(5) Contact with reality
(6) Sensorium and formal intelligence
(7) Insight and judgment

Observations under the first three headings at least will already have been made during the course of the general history and physical examination.

General appearance and behaviour
The patient's *appearance* may include evidence of subjective distress, as well as disturbance of thought, feeling, or behaviour of which he

may not be wholly aware. Such distress will presumably have been
mentioned in the statement of initial complaint when this has been
made, and may have been described as pain, exhaustion, uneasiness,
apprehension, fear, or a vague and general sense of malaise.

Useful information may be collected from the patient's *behaviour*
in the waiting room, his way of entering the room, his handshake
(willing, firm, timid, hesitant, sweaty), his direction of gaze, and
his clothes. By extension, further relevant points to be observed
are, who accompanies him, and, if he should be seen at home, the
style of surroundings he has there created for himself.

Talk
In recording observations about the patient's *manner and content
of talk*, attention should be paid to any special characteristics such
as slowing, flight of ideas, incoherence, circumstantiality or
evasiveness.

Subjective State
Disorder of mood requires assessment in the light of the patient's
life situation. *Anxiety* is the commonest of all unpleasant human
emotional experiences. It has been described as fear spread out
thin. *Depression* of mood, with sadness or foreboding which exceed
the patient's own capacity to justify or explain, or which may be
related to a general and intolerable deterioration in himself and the
world, may also be directly conveyed. Less often *unreasonable
exaltation* may be encountered; and the patient may show an elevation of mood which may shade off into frank *excitement*, clearly
abnormal and inappropriate to his circumstances.

Similarly his attitude to the consultation should have become
apparent by the time formal examination of mental state has been
reached. Such a mood and attitude as *suspicion*, or *bewilderment*,
will be noted here.

Content of Thought
This will include:

a) Disorders of thinking
b) Obsessive-compulsive phenomena
c) Ideas of reference and delusions
d) Other preoccupying themes.

a) Disorders of thinking include *thought block*, whereby the patient's capacity to maintain a train of thought is constantly interrupted, and other disorders described more fully in the chapter on *schizophrenia*. There is *retardation* when thinking is perceptibly slowed, and *acceleration* when it is speeded up to produce an effect of incoherence, with ideas tumbling over each other as the patient attempts to express them. *Flight of ideas*, with multiple associations, may have been revealed in talk by an incoherent jumble of rhymes or puns.

b) *Obsessive-compulsive ideas* emerge as repetitive preoccupations, which are recognized as unreasonable, but from which the patient cannot free himself. Such obsessive ideas, and actions dictated by them, form a particular group of distressing symptoms which patients may be prepared to discuss only when they feel that the doctor is at least familiar with the possibility of their occurrence, and sympathetic to their description.

c) *Ideas of reference* involve a disturbance of judgment and interpretation of external reality whereby the patient tends to relate external circumstances to himself, and so comes to believe that almost everything that happens has some special meaning directed towards him. This kind of disorder leads naturally to *delusions*, in explanation of the otherwise incomprehensible picture of the world which the patient obtains (see below).

d) Other *preoccupying themes* will be noted, such as grievances, detailed scrutiny of bodily function, religious fanaticisms, etc.

Contact with reality
This may be disturbed by *delusions, hallucinations* and *illusions*. A *delusion* is a false or mistaken belief, which has for the patient the force of conviction and is firmly held despite all evidence to the contrary. A *hallucination* is a perception through one of the senses, which does not correspond to any stimulus in the outside world; whereas an *illusion* is a perception which, although produced by an external stimulus, is misinterpreted by the patient in purely subjective terms.

Examples will make these three descriptive terms clear. If someone believes that he is being kept under constant observation by unknown enemies through radar or television, is having his food poisoned, or the air in his room contaminated by gas pumped through the ceiling, and cannot be induced to modify these beliefs, although they remain demonstrably untrue, then he is suffering from delusions. If he hears voices or sees visions, which no-one else can hear or see; or smells, for example, the gas which he believes to be entering the room, and if these experiences are in fact projections of his own fantasy, released by illness, then he is hallucinated. If, on the other hand, he mistakes his doctor or nurse for his father or mother, or for the devil come to take him away, then he is suffering from illusions which are being grafted on to the normal experience of seeing people, whose identity he misconstrues.

Delusions may be primary or secondary. Primary delusions are beliefs which arise spontaneously in the patient's mind, and which, although manifestly false, possess for the patient a degree of subjective certainty and conviction which nothing can alter. They carry a powerful feeling of *meaning* with them. Secondary delusions are equally mistaken beliefs of similar intensity and conviction, but are secondary in the sense that they represent the patient's attempt to find a reasonable explanation for other abnormal experiences: hallucinations, ideas of reference, or primary delusions, otherwise inexplicable.

A more diffuse disturbance of contact with reality is provided by a loss of the subjective conviction of the actual identity between one's self and one's body; or of the actuality of the rest of the world, normally taken for granted. Impairment in these fields is called depersonalization or derealization, respectively.

Sensorium and Formal Intelligence
Particular attention should be directed to recent and remote memory, to attention, concentration and grasp of problems and situations. The patient's ability to understand what is said to him, and to make appropriate response, although naturally subject to interference by hallucinations or delusions, ideas of reference or occasionally by obsessional ideas, will also come under this heading. Direct testing will elicit:
a) Orientation: for place, date and persons.
b) Memory:
(i) Remote past (this will have been tested in taking the preliminary history).
(ii) Recent past – some account of the last few days, checked by facts know to the examiner and by questions about world news. ·
(iii) Immediate retention – of a name, address, telephone number,

colour, name of a flower, objects shown, repetition of a series of digits forwards and backwards (normally six digits should be retained forwards and at least four reversed). A simple anecdote taking not more than one or two minutes to tell, can be repeated by the patient in his own words; and a formal sentence given to the patient for immediate repetition after learning. The traditional one is that of Babcock: 'One thing a nation must have to become rich and great is a good secure supply of wood'.

c) Attention: steady; or fluctuating, with distractibility.

d) Grasp of general information about life and current events.

e) Ability to perform simple calculations: change for small sums of money; serial subtraction of seven from 100 (100, 93, 86 . . . Note errors and time in seconds. Twenty seconds is a fast performance, thirty seconds average).

In these tests, observation is made not only of capacity to pass or fail, but also of consistency and especially jumbling in the results.

Insight and Judgment

Judgment of reasonable and realistic plans is noted. *Insight into illness* is noted by finding out whether the patient realizes that he is ill. If he does, is he able to accept his illness as responsible for the symptoms of which he complains, or does he consider, for example, that the persecution to which he is being subjected is the cause of his illness and not the outcome of it?

INFORMANTS

Any other information which may help to provide a many-sided picture of the patient and his difficulties in his world, should be welcomed. The implications as well as the actual statements in the letter of referral need attention. Offers of contact from school-teachers, employers, friends and neighbours may be relevant, always preserving the patient's confidentiality, the doctor listening but rarely talking.

Most of all, *other members of the immediate family* will be able to describe the patient's usual personality, how he has changed, and recent disorders in his behaviour which he may be minimizing or concealing. Disturbances may indeed be manifest in the relative, throwing doubt on who is truly to be regarded as the principal patient, or suggesting that the problem may be not so much illness or personal problem as an *interpersonal problem*, for example a marital unhappiness or disturbed parent-child relationship. The original 'indicated patient' may then turn out to be merely the first member of a disturbed family to reach the doctor. These matters may be made clearer by a *joint interview* of the people concerned, with observations of how they communicate with one another.

Evaluation of Findings

Examination of the mental state provides the raw material for the clinical study of personality in health and sickness, in terms of thought, feeling and behaviour. Their respective contribution to the total personality of an individual can conveniently be assessed in terms of three abstractions:

(1) Intelligence
(2) Emotional integration
(3) Instinctual drive

The purpose of abstractions of this kind is to provide a framework for clear description and understanding; just as concepts such as

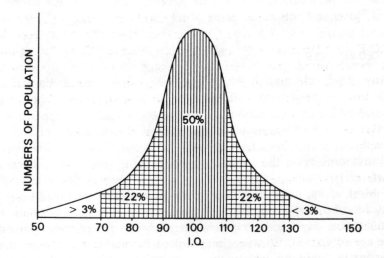

Intelligence distribution

length, breadth, thickness and mass are useful abstractions in the description of solid objects.

(1) *Intelligence* may be defined as the capacity to interpret experience, to learn from it, and to modify behaviour in the light of it. It can be measured with reasonable objectivity and accuracy, and is distributed throughout the population in a predictable way (see Figure).

The figure indicates the characteristic graph obtained when the numbers of any large random sample of a population are plotted against the intelligence levels of the individual members. It will be seen to be a symmetrical so-called normal curve of distribution. Taking the Intelligence Quotient of 100 as the standard mean level for the population, significant features are:

a) 50 per cent of the population have an I.Q. between 90 and 110.
b) A further 44 per cent are distributed symmetrically on either side of this, between 70 and 90 I.Q., and between 110 and 130 I.Q.
c) The remaining 6 per cent show an almost symmetrical distribution between subnormality (over 3 per cent below I.Q. 70) and outstanding intellectual endowment (less than 3 per cent over I.Q. 130). The slightly larger lower tail to the graph consists of cerebrally abnormal individuals (see Chapter 15).

As general guiding indications, successful completion of a professional training demands an I.Q. of not less than 120; 4 'O' levels in G.C.E., not less than 110; and a strictly average I.Q. of 100 equips its owner for no more than artisan occupation under supervision. Around I.Q. 80 only unskilled labouring can be managed, and at the level of about 70, employability is waning, and often only casual jobs are taken.

Formal tests of intelligence, normally administered by a clinical psychologist, are not based upon the subject's knowledge, but upon his ability to learn, and particularly to recognize and abstract logical patterns from experience, and to apply these patterns to the solution of problems. Tests of intelligence can be adjusted to the overall capacity of the subject under examination. The natural development of intelligence, like physical growth, is normally completed by about the age of sixteen. Wisdom, judgment and experience continue, but the innate capacity which has been achieved by the late teens or early twenties does not thereafter increase.

(2) *Emotion* may be defined as a combination of subjective feeling and objective physiological change. It provides the drive underlying behaviour, as well as the subjective response and accompaniment to experience. Emotional integration is not necessarily related to intelligence. This is exemplified in everyday experience by the fact that childishness in adults is not confined to the stupid.' Emotional integration can be regarded as the capacity of an individual to preserve a balance and consistency both in the way he feels about people and things, and what he does about them. It provides an index of the resilience and stability of a personality; and like intelligence it normally matures with age.

(3) *Instincts* are innate combinations of emotion and behaviour, directed towards goals unrelated to previous experience, which emerge spontaneously during the lifetime of an individual, and develop without having to be learned or acquired from outside. Strength of instinctual drive, like intelligence and capacity for emotional integration, varies from one individual to another; it is the principal determinant of that individual's basic level of persistence, flexibility, explosiveness, or stability of conduct.

The information provided by this clinical approach, using the relatively simple technique of history and examination outlined, at once supplies the doctor with a considerable insight into his patient's condition; he will be in a position to relieve the complaints of much of their affective burden, because he will have come far towards perceiving their genesis – and may well in the process have led his patient along with him to this discovery too.

The force of the indication for a full history in neurotic patients of varying grades of severity of illness is illustrated by brief consideration of three cases, all of which passed through the hands of general physicians whose knowledge and skill were unquestioned.

Case No. 1
A manual labourer in his late forties was referred to an outpatient department with hysterical spasm of the right hand. This was removed within half an hour by forceful suggestion and persuasion: the same evening the man was brought back into the hospital in a police ambulance with his throat cut. He had committed suicide. Subsequent inquiry revealed that he had for some months been becoming increasingly depressed, retarded and anxious; that his efficiency at work, which demanded a modicum of manual skill, had decreased to a point at which he was in grave danger of losing his job, and that this had further oppressed and worried him, as he had a wife and family dependent upon

him. The hysterical spasm had followed a trivial accident at work and represented the desperate temporary expedient of a simple man to stave off complete defeat and gain an honourable respite from the losing battle with a severe depression which he was endeavouring to right single-handed. The superficial cure had completed his undoing.

Case No. 2

A young ex-soldier of twenty-eight complained of eighteen months' history of anxiety, insomnia, headaches, backache and general fears for his health; the symptoms were the continuation of the illness for which he had been invalided from the Army eighteen months previously, after nine months in and out of hospital. He had done no work since his discharge. He was married with one child, a daughter aged two. This man's anxiety and headaches had begun during his wife's pregnancy. While in hospital undergoing investigation – which included lumbar puncture – he received news that his unit was being drafted overseas and that he had been taken off the draft. His reaction to this was a mixture of relief, guilt, and fear, the last emotion crystallizing around the possible result and significance of the lumbar puncture which his fellow patients assured him meant that the doctors suspected syphilis. He had been unfaithful to his wife once, during her pregnancy, and this increased both his guilt and fear of venereal disease. The reaction of certain psychopaths who happened to be in the ward at that time was to congratulate him upon what they insisted must have been his deliberate astuteness in dodging the draft on medical grounds, and to infer that there must be little he didn't know about malingering – unless of course he really had got syphilis. He had been as discomfited by their congratulations as he was alarmed and shamed by their speculations. Not simply his physical health but his personal integrity seemed compromised and in question: he had remained anguished and in doubt, and his anxiety, superficially focused on the possible implications and result of lumbar puncture, in fact extended deeply through his whole personality and undermined it. Once this became apparent, together with its contributory causes, he improved rapidly with comparatively superficial psychotherapy, resumed work, and regained sexual potency, the loss of which during his illness he had not even dared to mention to a doctor before. A year later he remained well and at work.

Case No. 3

A spinster of forty-eight who had nursed her invalid mother for many years prior to the latter's death from carcinoma of the breast, herself developed a lump in the breast which for some time she feared to reveal to her doctor. Having ultimately undergone biopsy at another hospital she was informed that a second operation would be necessary and would take the form of a 'deeper cut'. On recovery from the anaesthetic on the second occasion she discovered that she had undergone a radical mastectomy and became increasingly depressed, paranoid, and deluded, convinced that her 'inside had been removed, womanhood taken away, no longer a person at all, converted into a living corpse . . .'. She was transferred to an inpatient psychiatric unit, the diagnosis being severe depressive reaction with secondary paranoid features and hysterical overlay. The patient remained psychotic for two months but ultimately recovered though still attending for follow-up and support.

During follow-up and support her constant lament in retrospect has been 'Why didn't anyone have the time to listen to my fears or explain what they were going to do to me, before the operation . . . ?'

These three cases could easily be multiplied. All have one essential feature in common. In every one the vitally essential information was there, available to any examiner 'with the time' to seek it out; in every one failure to do so had resulted in a greater or less degree of disaster for the patients; in the first death; in the second, at least eighteen months' invalidism and loss of regular work; in the third, an explosive psychotic illness complicating recovery from a major operation.

The inference from all this is not simply that more research, and more appropriately trained consultants, specialists, and ancillary workers in this branch of medicine are required, although this is undoubtedly true. What is far more important is that doctors in general should have an adequate basic grasp of the part played by psychological factors in everyday illness, and the part which they themselves can play in recognizing and treating this, in precisely the same way that they are expected to recognize and treat the occurrence of medical, surgical and obstetric conditions in their daily practice.

Most important of all is for every doctor to accept and understand that psychological illness is not a thing apart; it is fundamentally an aspect of all illness, and the psychological component of any illness requires the appropriate degree of attention if adequate care is ever to be given to any patient.

Chapter 3

Personality Development

The clinical approach already described presents the physician with a cross-section of the patient's total personality in terms of the three abstractions outlined: intelligence, emotional integration, and instinctual drive (p. 36). Its effective interpretation demands an understanding of the development of personality from birth onwards, in the same terms. This development could be described in a number of different ways, and from different points of view: the present account emphasizes the inner experiences of the individual, and is therefore necessarily speculative in places, especially when describing early infancy.

Consciousness, defined as the total of subjective awareness at any moment, can for practical purposes be assumed to begin at birth. The infant's first response to this beginning takes a form which will always later be associated with over-whelming emotion, usually of a disagreeable kind. In fact, he cries.

What is happening at this instant is that the baby's consciousness is being flooded with signals or sense impressions through every receptor channel between the periphery of his body and his cerebral cortex. Such signals from his eyes, his ears, his nose, and the whole sensory surface of his body, together with those related to position sense in his muscles and joints, are combining to flood consciousness with a bombardment of incoming stimuli which are as yet totally unrelated to each other, and in no way integrated to make any recognizable assimilable pattern of experience. It is the progressive integration and assimilation of such incoming stimuli, their correlation with each other, and the acquisition of patterns of experience made up of groups or sets of such stimuli having a constant relationship to each other, that forms the whole basis of learning, and of the development of the mental life of the individual.

There is evidence that this process is not only difficult and extremely complicated, but may well be in one sense, disagreeable. Professor J. Z. Young, writing of the development of what he calls 'rules for establishing certainty in the brain', describes one source of knowledge about this in a particularly vivid and interesting way.

'We have no means of examining and recording all that happens in the brains of babies and very young children. But we can learn a great deal that is helpful from the reports of people with certain rather rare forms of blindness who, though born blind, have later been operated on and receive their sight. This is a specially favourable opportunity by which we may examine, as it were, phases of childhood being passed through in a person who can talk . . .

'Such a patient on opening his eyes for the first time gets little or no enjoyment; indeed, he finds the experience painful. He reports only a spinning mass of lights and colours. He proves to be quite unable to pick out objects by sight, to recognize what they are, or to name them. He has no conception of a space with objects in it, although he knows all about objects and their names by touch . . .

'Unless he is quite clever and very persistent he may never learn to make use of his eyes at all. At first he only experiences a mass of colour but gradually he learns to distinguish shapes. When shown a patch of one colour placed on another he will quickly see that there is a difference between the patch and its surroundings. What he will not do is to recognize that he has seen that particular shape before, nor will he be able to give it its proper name.

'For example, one man when shown an orange a week after beginning to see said that it was gold. When asked "What shape is it?" he said "Let me touch it and I will tell you!" After doing so he said it was an orange. Then he looked long at it and said, "Yes, I can see that it is round." Shown next a blue square, he said it was blue and round. A triangle he also described as round. When the angles were pointed out to him he said, "Ah, yes, I understand now, one can *see* how they feel."

'For many weeks and months after beginning to see, the person can only with great difficulty distinguish between the simplest shapes, such as a triangle and a square. If you ask him how he does it, he may say, "Of course if I look carefully I see that there are three sharp turns at the edge of the one patch of light, and four on the other. . . ." If you show him the two the next day he will be quite unable to say which is a triangle and which a square. . . .

However such people can gradually learn; if sufficiently encouraged they may after some years develop a full visual life and be able even to read.

'It takes at least a month to learn the names of even a few objects. Gradually the patient leaves out the laborious counting of the corners and comes to identify things so quickly that, as in an ordinary person, the process by which he does so is not apparent. So it is not that all along the eyes or brain were incapable of acting normally. What these people lack is the store of rules in the brain, rules usually learnt by the long years of exploration with the eyes during childhood. They have no models with which to compare the input, no mould or filter that can be used to select the significant features of visual experience and produce appropriate words and other motor responses. A normal person learns the rules of seeing by connecting some parts of the sensory input with motor acts that lead to satisfaction, for instance, naming and the fulfilment of communication.'

So much for the difficulties of integrating experience; and from neurophysiology we know something of the kind of brain activity which is necessary to master this complex procedure. Electro-encephalographic recordings of action currents in the brain of a baby show that, during waking life, the activity of various parts of the brain is largely unco-ordinated. The number, variety and amplitude of the various waves recorded on the electroencephalogram, in terms both of wave length and frequency, are exceedingly complicated at this stage of life. When the baby is asleep, the majority of neurones appear to be undergoing a synchronous pulsation, and while it is true that the brain can be regarded as resting during this period, it is probably also then that the assimilated patterns of the waking period of activity are being stored and integrated.

As the child grows up, and becomes by stages an adult, the overall change is recorded by the electroencephalogram as a simplification of waking brain wave patterns; a simplification which seems to be connected with a greater degree of integration and co-ordination of activity in the various parts of the brain. The complexity and stress implicit in this theory of the kind of activity required of the brain in performing its initial integration of order out of apparent chaos during the first few weeks and months of life, provides one possible explanation of why the new-born baby needs to spend so great a proportion of the daily twenty-four hours isolated from the bombardment of sensory experience in sleep. New-born babies require as much as twenty hours' sleep in twenty-four, and can therefore be thought of as being exposed to the bombard-ment for about four hours, while resting and integrating the effects of each successive bombardment in preparation for the next, for the remaining twenty.

In effect, what the baby is doing is making a picture of the world and his place in it, out of this continual bombardment of sensory experience to which he is subjected during his waking hours; and out of the constant and progressive sorting and assimilation of this experience, he becomes able within a matter of weeks or months to make some vitally important discoveries about himself and the world about him.

EMERGENCE OF SELF

Probably his first recognition is that there is a part of life and experience which is permanently with him, and which later still he comes to recognize is actually part of him; and another part, con-stantly fluctuating and changing, which is in some way beyond and outside him. The distinction which the child may be imagined to be making at this stage, is between what is 'me' and what is 'not-me'. In this context, it is essential to remember that any description of the beginning of experience and of its integration in the developing mind of the infant, conveyed in words, is bound to contain and imply at least one potentially important source of error; namely the implication that babies think, and understand their thoughts, in words.

As adults we tend to take verbal thinking for granted. It has to be remembered that a child does not learn the use of words, as complex flexible tools for symbolic communication, until he begins to learn to talk. All his thinking up to this time is non-verbal, and it is a striking reflection that a great deal of what is probably the most difficult brain work that an individual ever has to do, is done at a time in his life when he has not acquired that system of communi-cation and symbolic expression of his thoughts, without which later thinking would appear to be almost impossible.

In fact a great deal of this early and integrative work which lays the foundations for mental life, appears to be done at an uncon-scious level. And as we shall see later, it is characteristic of unconscious mental processes that they are either entirely non-verbal, or make a very different use of symbols, including words, from that which is made in conscious thought. But while the baby has no words for the 'me'/'not-me' division which he makes, it is the first and most fundamental division of many which will finally establish his picture of the world.

The most important single aspect of the part of experience which is 'not-me', comes eventually to be recognized as a constant element against an inconstant background; and this constant element is ultimately recognized as the child's first concept of the mother as another person, instinctively accepted as the indispensable link between 'me' and everything else.

This relationship is a fundamental one which has to occur if the child is to develop normally, although it can be made with any other individual who occupies the mother's place in the early life of the child. It is the mother's own special relationship to the child and her personal feelings about him which tend to make her the ideal person to fulfil this role.

One effect of the 'me'/'not-me' division is that the child comes to realize, still without the ability to conceive of this in words, that he is both dependent upon and at the mercy of his external environment. His mother is therefore not only emotionally indispensable, but his sole consistent source of physical comfort and affection. It is in this way that what is sometimes called the child's sense of insecurity comes to be balanced by his confidence in, and reliance upon his mother. But even this most early and fundamentally necessary mental adjustment is not without its difficulties. For the mother is not only the sole and essential source of comfort, satisfaction, warmth and protection; she is also the only apparent originator of frustration of any kind. It is she who picks up the child, cuddles and feeds him. But it is also she who puts him down, or leaves him, or fails to gratify him instantly on every occasion on which he may feel and express his needs with a cry.

In fact of course this frustration is as essential a part of his experience of life, as are the more agreeable aspects of it. Life, as a matter of practical experience, abounds with frustrations, as well as with opportunities; and it is only by meeting them early, continuing to meet them, and discovering within ourselves and our relationship with others some way of contending with them, that we can ultimately achieve any degree of emotional security. But nevertheless this aspect of the growing up process is an unwelcome and disagreeable one while it is occurring, and the child probably feels no gratitude to the mother for her inevitable part in it.

Thus it comes about, that even while he is still physically and emotionally entirely dependent upon his mother, the child is bound to experience frustration as well as gratification at her hands. His reaction to this is simple and quite unmistakable; he both loves and hates his mother. He loves her for all that she does for him, and he hates her for all that inevitably she cannot do, or fails to do. The discovery that one can entertain two such intensely conflicting and therefore painfully antagonistic feelings for the same person, a discovery which probably takes place somewhere between the fourth and sixth months of life, has been postulated as marking the stage of emotional development at which it is first possible to feel moods of happiness and depression, as opposed to simple reactions of satisfaction or displeasure. To have become thus capable of experiencing joy and sadness is to have taken a long and important step forward upon the road of life.

IMPORTANCE OF RELATIONSHIP WITH MOTHER

The vital importance of the mother in the life of her child, by the time this relationship has endured for six months of the child's life, has gained increasing recognition during the past fifty years, largely due to the work of pioneer psychiatrists such as Dr John Bowlby. It has been vividly illustrated by Dr Rene Spitz in New York and Drs James and Joyce Robertson of the Tavistock Institute of Human Relations in London.

Dr Bowlby reported on small children removed to institutions, often with very lonely and inhumane conditions, describing the distress and withdrawal clearly amounting to a kind of severe depression. Periods of months were thought to lead to permanent changes in the personality, including a loss of the capacity to love. Later writers linked this with the frequency of broken homes in the childhood of psychopathic personalities, to propagate the view that 'maternal deprivation' was a major cause of irreversible emotional crippling and crime. It can now be seen that the claims for long-term effects were far ahead of the evidence, and even during short separations, there have been few studies which could pinpoint the factors which distressed the child, whether separation from the mother, or other disturbing features of the transfer to an institution – the unfamiliar surroundings, strange noises, different routines, staff changes, and the fact that the children were sometimes ill and in pain.

Dr Spitz made a memorable film, *Grief: a peril in infancy*, a documentary report of the effect upon infants of prolonged separation from the mother, or mother substitute, during the first year of life. It observes the development of reversible patterns of what is clearly intensely depressed behaviour, during the absence of the mother lasting up to three months, and of more serious symptoms approaching psychotic intensity and accompanied by grave mental and physical retardation during longer or permanent absence of the mother. Some examples from its general content, selected from a review published by the Health Education Council of America, should make this clear.

A baby loses her mother
A child, Jane, noted for her good relations with her mother is shown greeting the male observer. She is alert and active and smiles happily when approached. The next scene is taken a few weeks later, one week after Jane's mother is forced to leave her in hospital. The approach of the observer now elicits bewilderment, then disappointment, and finally weeping. Titles explain that Jane's apathy and weeping last throughout the whole three month period of her mother's absence.

Two further instances emphasize the consistency of the pattern. A responsive, happy seven months old child is shown actively enjoying the visit of the observer. A few weeks after separation from the mother, the same child is apathetic and uninterested in the observer's advances. At a later visit, the child, by now eleven months old, lies dejected and withdrawn and is even less responsive and interested. When approached, the child begins to weep, and although reassurance silences the weeping to some extent, the child's facial expression remains impassive and cheerless. The departure of the observer precipitates another outbreak of weeping and distress. A third child, three months after separation from his mother, hides his face and curls up in a withdrawn attitude.

Babies reared without mothers
If the separation of mother and infant lasts longer than three months, the child becomes apathetic, withdrawn, and no longer weeps but now wails thinly. Lasting personality changes may result. Representative cases were selected from ninety-one children at a foundling home, all of whom lost their mothers during their fourth month of life. At the home they have been given excellent hygienic, nutri-

tional, and medical care: but no one individual has had the time to give each baby a mother's love. Six children are shown, ranging from eight to fifteen months in age; not one is able to sit or stand. Among these, an eight months old pair of twins show retarded behaviour; one behaves like a three month old infant, and the other is completely passive. Other babies show bizarre movements which resemble those of children with psychotic disturbances. A fifteen months old infant, who appears to be about three months of age, is an example of these children who fail to develop properly and who easily succumb to disease or intercurrent infection.

In children somewhat older, who had been sent to institutions between the ages of $1\frac{1}{2}$ and $2\frac{1}{2}$ years, Robertson described in detail stages of protest, despair and denial, as follows:

'In the phase of *protest*, the newly separated young child commonly protests bitterly against the loss of his mother and seeks by shouting and crying to regain her; he may resist the attentions of nurses. Then, after a few hours or a few days, protest gives way to *despair*: the child no longer shouts and cries, but is quiet and uncomplaining, maybe grizzles. If reunited at this point he may turn from his mother in anger, and be insecure and difficult to manage for a long time afterwards. If the separation goes on for long enough in a setting where caretakers change and there is no opportunity for stable relationships, despair is succeeded by *denial* (sometimes called *detachment*). In this final phase the child is superficially bright and indiscriminately sociable, and is so detached from meaningful relationships that he appears unaffected by the comings and goings of his visiting parents or by changes of staff'.

The Robertsons are now renowned for further studies in which children were studied during excellent foster-care, in fact in the Robertsons' own home, the observations being made into the series of films *Young children in brief separation*. Their results are very different:

'Our study suggests that, when separated, young children continue to offer cues for care and interaction in expectation of responses similar to those they have known at home; and that the extent to which they are able to cope with the loss of the mother will be influenced by the ability of the caretakers to recognize and respond to the cues that are offered.

'Thus John, who was put into a residential nursery, tried repeatedly to attach himself to one or other of the many nurses; it was only after they had each failed to respond that he turned away in acute distress succeeded by apathetic withdrawal. But when the four fostered children reached out in a similar tentative way this was responded to by the fully available foster mother. This relationship held the children emotionally, and they continued to function well. Although anxious because of the loss of the mother, they were not overwhelmed as John was. They did not suffer trauma.

'The fostered children's experience of good mothering was maintained throughout the separation; therefore at reunion each of them returned warmly to the mother with the expectation of good mothering. But because John had been deprived of responsive mothering care he was hostile at reunion'.

These studies show vividly that children need the maintenance of the emotional relationships with their mothers or of a similar substitute, as much as they need food, shelter or any other necessity of life, for their full development. They also reveal poignantly how closely akin extreme grief in an infant is to similar emotion in an adult, in its ultimate expression.

EFFECTS OF THREATS AND FRUSTRATIONS

Of course the normal child tends to escape these misfortunes, although the importance of separation from the mother in infancy has only been fully appreciated from the scientific standpoint in the last twenty-five years. But the continuing pressure of the outside world upon the life of the child nevertheless produces, as we have seen, other and more manageable frustrations of which probably the next most important one is the emergence of the father in a necessarily dual and divided role. It is this which forms the basis of what Freud came to call the Oedipus complex, and which he postulated as the major source of potential neuroses in both sexes.

In effect, the young child is apt to be faced with what is for him an insoluble emotional conflict between his jealousy of the father as a rival, and his awareness of dependence upon him as the stable background of family life. The natural outcome of the child's jealousy, and sense of his own comparative inadequacy as a rival with his father, are aggressive wishes and feelings directed against the father, when the father's influence and claims upon the mother come into conflict with the child's own desire for her exclusive attention and concern. Moreover these powerful, hostile feelings are not only forbidden in the child's mind, but are also opposed by the love, respect, and trust which he normally feels for his father as a person. Indeed if he is a boy his natural desire will be to model himself upon his father and to be like him; and he is therefore once again faced with a conflict between resenting and loving the same person, between holding that person up as a wonderful and admired model for his own emulation on the one hand, and yet at times wishing the overthrow or disappearance of this model so that he can himself take his place.

The conflict occasioned by loving your rival, and by feeling that your happiness and security are threatened by jealousy of your best friend, is a theme whose poignancy endures throughout adult life and is a favoured motif in literature and drama; and this reflection of the earliest and most acute emotional problems of childhood upon the wider screen of adult experience, is but one example of the way in which powerful feelings associated with our earliest and perhaps least integrated emotional experiences tend to influence all our later interests, hopes and fears. For when the child first experiences this conflict of feeling about his father he is in the very earliest years of his life, at a time when there is no possible solution of it which can prove finally or decisively satisfactory to him one way or another. Nor is it something he can think over to himself or discuss with other people; for once again we have to remember that he has no words either to symbolize his thoughts or to convey them to others.

This constellation of feelings and ideas with a strong emotional charge, closely connected both with the father's role and with the child's feelings about it, and about his own position in the whole situation, provides a vivid example of overwhelmingly intense experience. Experience of this degree of emotional intensity could in fact be a very threatening factor in the child's development, just as we have seen is the case with separation from mothering. But there is a natural mechanism which develops in human beings along with their capacity to experience emotional stress, whose function it is to prevent such emotional stress from overwhelming the integration and development of their personality. The first person to discover and describe this mechanism fully in understandable terms, was Sigmund Freud. This is not the least of his claims to serious attention in the study of psychology.

LATER CHILDHOOD

The period of infancy normally ends somewhere between the fourth and fifth year, and from this time onwards the child increasingly develops a capacity to make his own relationships of an enduring kind with the outside world and the people who inhabit it. While he is to some extent still contained, so to speak, within the emotional aura of his mother's life, and will so remain until he is at least seven or eight years old, he can now go forth and meet other people, accepting his relationship with them on the basis of whatever relationship he has so far achieved with his parents. He goes to school, he meets and plays with other children, he shares the wider frustrations and responsibilities of growing up.

Whereas previously he has been an entirely self-centred and emotionally explosive individual, now he becomes more and more an individual existing in a community, and taking some of his satisfaction as well as giving some of his efforts in relation to his place in this community. It is during this stage of his life that he lays the foundations of formal learning which will later equip him for all the abstract problems of adult existence.

By contrast with the explosiveness of infancy, there is a curious stability and plasticity throughout this stage of human development. This lasts until about the age of nine to eleven, when a second great wave of change begins to sweep over the individual. This is the onset of physiological sexual maturity. The sexual instinct, present from birth but hitherto existing in a more vague, diffuse and but dimly perceived form, and lacking until now the full development both of a physical means for its expression, and the stronger drive towards such expression to which this bodily development gives rise, now gradually comes to dominate the emotional development of the child who has begun to be a child no longer.

ADOLESCENCE

When the individual reaches this stage of development, a whole avalanche of increased tension and conflict floods his life. Without being fully aware of it, he experiences again, and now in an intensified form, all the old feelings of rivalry, insecurity and aggression of infancy, with the parents in their old roles as well as in the newer ones with which adolescence confronts him.

Young people at this stage of development are apt to be particularly critical of all the things that their parents have most wanted to impress upon them as they grow up; and they may even seem to the parents to take delight in following the opposite line on everything which the parents have felt was important in their upbringing. The child of strict churchgoers may go through a period, at least, of proclaiming himself an atheist; the free thinker's daughter may want to become a nun. To the children these decisions represent passionately sincere and obviously necessary gestures; but they are gestures which all too often strike the parents as merely wantonly contrary.

This can be for all concerned a most turbulent and unhappy time. The individual feels himself to be beyond the old safe, secure, and at least partly explored boundaries of childhood experience, and to be venturing into a no-man's land leading to adult independence and power which still seem magically remote: and yet he is without the confidence or experience of adult life from which he feels himself in some way excluded, and which therefore he tends to envy and to resent.

The period of rebellion and hostility against authority in general, and parents in particular, is part of a natural and indeed an inevitable stage of development. Adolescents themselves are partly aware of the considerable practical disadvantage which surrounds them at this stage of their lives. In one way they may be likened to displaced persons in a strange land. The gates of childhood are closing behind them, but they have no passport to adult independence and prestige. They stand, uneasy and aggressive for a time, in a kind of no-man's land between frontiers. Their parents no longer seem the powerful figures that dominated childhood, and on whom they relied both for protection and for infallibility; and yet if they cannot accept their parents, still less can they wholly accept themselves.

They are aware of developing emotions with a consciously sexual flavour whose intensity excites and disturbs them, making them both self-conscious and apt to be resentful of the adults whom they half envy and half admire. And for all this they tend to blame their unfortunate parents, now stripped of most of the prestige once accorded to them, and now seeming to be obstacles to the freedom which the adolescent passionately desires, but still partly fears.

Parents now stand for all that has to be challenged and criticized rather than obeyed; and yet in many ways parents are needed more at this time than they will ever be needed again.

Many people find themselves relatively unable to remember this period of their lives in any detail. For those who can remember it, the memory is seldom particularly happy, although all human beings, protected to some extent from too much overt disturbance occasioned by resurrection of past shames, uncertainties, fears, disappointments or humiliations, tend to remember no more than they can bear. The characteristics of the average adolescent, viewed objectively and from without, can be related to those processes in the development of his personality which we have just been examining.

The normal adolescent is comparatively indifferent to children, essentially divided in his attitude towards grown-up people, and alternately fierce and tender towards others like himself. There is, however, a tendency to form defensive bonds and alliances between young people of this age, recognized in our society by interminable discussions about the problems of 'teenagers', and the recognition of their somewhat prickly and sensitive identification with each other as a group. They tend to be bewildered by their own feelings, both by their intensity and by the moods which they produce, and for much of the time are thrown back upon introspection and fantasy. This is in fact a chaotic period of development, and approaches more closely what we shall later understand as the pattern of neurotic illness, than any other period in the life of the normal individual.

Adolescence is in fact always a period of turbulent emotion, sometimes of disturbed behaviour, and a time when love, tolerance, and imaginative understanding were never more in demand and yet never harder wholly to accept. This is not of course to say that normal adolescence is a period of unrelieved gloom or despair, but rather that the many consolations, pleasures and excitements of these remarkable years tend to belong either to what has been brought over from childhood, or to what is hopefully anticipated in maturity.

MATURITY

With the ending of adolescence, somewhere between the seventeenth and nineteenth year or thereabouts, the period of entering upon full maturity has begun. In the normal individual all the patterns of instinctive behaviour with their attendant emotions which will characterize his further development have by now made their appearance, and despite the increasing complexity of the struggle for existence in the outer world, the most explosive phases of adjustment to his inner life, to himself and his relationship to others, will by now have been completed. By now the patterns which have been laid down for dealing with success and failure, the capacities which have been formed for loving or hating, trusting or suspecting, accepting or rejecting other people, are in essence already formed. They remain influences rather than absolute determinant factors, and modification of course is always possible; but such modification is never simply a matter of reason and intelligence in the light of experience; it depends far more upon the extent to which new emotional responses, with the attendant risk of new and perhaps painful adjustments, can be tolerated within the personality of the individual concerned.

It is a matter of objective observation and clinical experience that it is always extremely difficult for an individual to alter or give up a habit of emotional response which has become ingrained in the most sensitive and formative years of childhood, in the course of the child's relationship with those most close to him. This can be exemplified by the case of a child whose relationship with his father has been unhappy, whose need and desire to respect, admire, and love the father has been thwarted and replaced by resentment, jealousy, or a sense of betrayal. Such a person will find even when he has left childhood behind, that every relationship with older men, or those charged with authority, is for him an exceedingly difficult and challenging one. Sometimes a lifetime will not be enough to enable such a person to make a better adjustment to this emotional predicament, which burdens him constantly with the threat and the shadow of far-off, half-remembered days, whose present impact he may well deny.

FORMATION OF NEUROTIC PATTERNS

The tendency to build up patterns of behaviour during emotional development, and to be influenced by them repetitively and without consciousness of their origin from that time on, is essentially a normal one. But when these patterns happen to be particularly morbid or unsuccessful they form the basis for all the wide and protean manifestations of what are called neurotic illness or neurotic patterns of activity.

A sound and helpful way of regarding neurosis, and the neurotic patient, is to regard neurosis as the perpetuation of patterns of response which have started by being abnormally unsuccessful, and have produced subsequently a series of increasingly intolerable situations with correspondingly intolerable emotional experiences, to which the patient's desperate and increasingly unsuccessful response is in fact a further repetition of the original pattern. Adolescence is in one way a reliving of the explosiveness of infancy under new circumstances; the extent to which the patterns of infancy are completely repeated is the extent to which adolescence is turbulent, unhappy, and neurotic. The extent to which this chaotic but necessarily formative period leads to the emergence of newer and more flexible patterns of behaviour, determines the success with which the individual emerges from adolescence into maturity.

It is necessary for the doctor always to remember this similarity between neurotic behaviour and normal behaviour, as well as its difference. When in a difficult, threatening, and provocative environment the average individual contrives to remain reasonably happy and moderately stable for much of the time, it is because the basic patterns of behaviour which he has acquired during childhood and adolescence are reasonably sound, and because his capacity to modify them is not abnormally limited. This is one way of expressing the concept of emotional maturity; namely as a combination of reasonably sound, stable, and efficient patterns of behaviour with sufficient flexibility and resilience to enable them to be modified in the light of experience during adult life.

While there is ample evidence, as we shall see later, that the capacity for achieving emotional maturity is at least to some extent innate and constitutional, in precisely the same way as is the capacity for achieving comparable maturity of intellectual development, the actual variations in degree and nature of the patterns displayed during the individual's lifetime are of course largely reactive to the experiences which that lifetime has produced. Of all these experiences, those during the first decade and a half will always remain the most important in their influence upon the life of the individual.

THE ROLE OF INTELLIGENCE

Whereas objective measurement of emotional maturity is a difficult and disputed task, objective measurement of intellectual maturity is comparatively straightforward. The development of emotional maturity and of intelligence, although interrelated, and proceeding side by side during infancy, childhood and adolescence, are by no means identical, and can be separately studied. One of the first attempts to measure the faculty of intelligence objectively was made in the early part of the twentieth century by Binet in Paris.

This approach was founded on the concept of intelligence as the capacity to modify behaviour successfully in response to changing situations, and to learn by experience. Binet's technique involved setting children a variety of problems and puzzles to solve, with assessment in terms of *mental age*. A child who just solved the problems typically solved by four-year olds would have a mental age of four, but if he failed these and only passed those usually soluble by three-year olds, he would have a mental age of three, being retarded by one year. In development through childhood, the ratio of mental age over chronological age tends to remain constant, whether in slow or quick developers, and when multiplied by 100 is widely quoted as the intelligence quotient or I.Q., with a statistical mean of 100.

Over the age of sixteen, when the development of intelligence has flattened out, the figure indicating the measure of intelligence in relation to the norm in the population of that age, has to be drawn up differently. The average score for all people is called 100, and mathematical adjustment is used to fix other scores along the distribution curve. As described in the last chapter, the middle 50 per cent of all scores in the population are said to be between I.Q.s 90 and 110, and using the mathematical and statistical properties of the distribution curve, all test scores can be converted to I.Q. figures.

A full intelligence test, such as the frequently used Wechsler Adult Intelligence Scale, has a battery of subscales, setting a variety of different tasks, more or less evidently related to basic intelligence. Some are abstract problems to be solved with spatial skills, such as the tests of digit symbol, picture completion, block design, picture arrangement and object assembly, these five being conventionally combined in the 'performance score'. Others emphasize language, and tests called information, comprehension, similarities, digit span, vocabulary and arithmetic make up the 'verbal score'. Tables allow for combining these scores into a full scale I.Q.

The immediate fact to be grasped about intelligence is that it is not a static quality, but a dynamic one. To use a simple analogy, it is more like the potential rate of acceleration of a motor car, than its top speed, or the speed at which the car happens to be going at the time of measurement. Such rate of acceleration is always related directly to power; and if we know the power of an engine we can make a reasonable estimate of its potential performance, whether or not that potential is currently in use.

The analogy of a car can be taken further to illustrate the actual development of intelligence in a human being. We can imagine the car starting from rest and accelerating steadily up to its maximum speed; this it maintains for a considerable time, and then with wear and tear and age the speed gradually declines. Finally some vital part of the mechanism wears out or breaks down, and the car stops.

The period of acceleration from rest corresponds to the development of intelligence from birth to about the age of sixteen; thereafter, although judgment, experience, and the wisdom that results from their combination will continue to develop, the effective level of innate intelligence tends to remain constant, until in the latter half of life it gradually, although at first almost imperceptibly, declines. This decline tends in practice to be offset in terms of individual performance, and in the assessment of the casual observer, by that accumulation of judgment, experience and wisdom which characterize the later stages of life. But a decline in innate intelligence it nevertheless remains, and as such it can be detected by suitably sensitive methods of testing, long before its more manifest appearance in the evening of life.

During life, just as a car's speed may fluctuate and respond either to the control of the driver or the efficiency of the engine – faltering for example with dirty fuel or a defective electrical system – so an individual's intellectual performance will be affected both by the degree to which emotional factors influence his inclination or capacity to use his intelligence, as well as by the health and structural integrity of his brain and nervous system.

NORMAL OLD AGE

In cognitive matters, the decline in intelligence has been noted. At the same time alertness is in eclipse, and the ability to consider several complex matters at once. Memory begins to fail in efficiency, especially the registration and recall of new experiences, and the learning of completely new fields of knowledge and new kinds of intellectual activity is made increasingly difficult by faulty recall of what has finally, after many trials, been committed to memory. The old person lives on intellectual capital from the past.

Emotionally, maximum stability has been achieved, until the cerebral changes of late senility undermine it again, bringing back the lability, tetchiness and tears of 'second childhood'. Changes of settled viewpoints are not now to be expected, and interests become limited, horizons nearer. The world may revolve around small numbers of acquaintances and family, and spells of relative inactivity alone may take up much of the day. The old person may become a *laudator temporis acti*, limit his interests to the decline of standards in the modern world, his faltering health and the possibility of his becoming destitute, at least the last two of these being frequently realistic. Sexual activity declines steadily, although it can be kept in being remarkably successfully by unbroken practice dating from younger times.

Retirement from work may be very unsettling, and in the absence of preparation, and in people with limited resources of personality but with much invested in work to the neglect of home life, the complete change in way of life and personal relationships may precipitate mental illness. The preventive is richness of life and interests outside work, and niches where the retired man is still welcomed and needed, and so is himself satisfied in the later years.

The experience of being widowed is more shattering than retirement, being usually unexpected, rupturing relationships of far deeper moment to the survivor, and leaving him perhaps in complete emotional isolation. In addition to the tragedy and distress, it is followed in a number of cases by psychiatric morbidity and even death.

The decline in physical and mental vigour together is but one more instance of the indissoluble inter-relationship between all aspects of living, from the biochemical to the personal, which appears to be a fundamental condition of human existence. Acceptance and understanding of the implications of this interrelationship are therefore indispensable elements in the training of a doctor.

THE PSYCHODYNAMIC HYPOTHESIS

A key to the mental processes whereby the explosiveness of infancy is succeeded, first by the relative docility of childhood, then by the turbulence of adolescence, and finally by the degree of intellectual, emotional, and behavioural integration and maturity characteristic of the normal adult, is provided by the concepts of *repression* and the *unconscious mind*.

An important tenet of psycho-dynamic theory is that childhood experiences provide in simplified form a preparation for all the later emotional events of adult life, including for example such disturbing feelings as sexual jealousy, and the conflict between loving and hating the same person, to which such jealousy can give rise. When conflict of this kind reaches a pitch of intensity sufficiently unbearable to threaten the entire mental and emotional stability of the person experiencing it, it may disappear from consciousness entirely by a process of automatic and involuntary forgetting first described by Freud, who gave it the name of repression.

This particular kind of forgetting is postulated as a normal mental function, both in childhood, and to a lesser extent, in normal adult life. It results in the forgotten material being no longer available to direct recall, nor even represented in consciousness by the vaguest awareness that it ever existed. A constellation of ideas, surrounding an experience with intense emotional charge, which has been repressed in this way, is called a complex; a term borrowed by Freud from Jung, who was at the time his pupil.

By involving a most skilful method of making use of people's capacity to retrace ideas by means of their associations, Freud was able to demonstrate that much of this forgotten material was in fact still present in the minds of adults, although no longer capable of direct recall, nor normally recognized or experienced in any way. The area of mind where this material lay buried Freud named the unconscious. He held therefore that there are at least three main levels of mental life which may contain ideas and feelings of importance in determining behaviour; consciousness, which is a reflection of everything of which we are immediately aware; pre-consciousness, which is the reservoir of all that is accessible to voluntary recall, and contains therefore everything which we can remember; and finally the unconscious area of mental life. The unconscious area includes both the origins of instinctual drives, which ultimately reach consciousness in the form of impulses to behave in certain ways, and repressed complexes, which may influence feeling and action without ever themselves regaining consciousness. They do this by creating emotional tension, whose origin remains unconscious.

Broadly speaking, it is evident that the effect that will be produced when a repressed complex is stirred by some event in the conscious experience of the individual which has similar associations, will be the production of emotions appropriate to the complex, and therefore probably highly unpleasant or unbearable.

Since the most common reasons for repression are that the repressed material has been charged with feelings either of intense hostility or guilt, or intense fear or anxiety, these are likely to be the feelings aroused when a complex is activated. What happens therefore is that unpleasant feelings are aroused, but because of the effectiveness of the repression of the actual experience with which they were originally associated, the person concerned remains completely unaware of their source. It is this flooding of consciousness with highly unpleasant feelings, together with their emotional or physical repercussions, which gives rise to many of the symptoms of mental illness or psychosomatic disorder with which psychiatry is concerned.

Nevertheless repression is a normal homeostatic mechanism, whereby psychological equilibrium is maintained, by the exclusion from consciousness and preconsciousness of overwhelmingly threatening or disturbing memories. During infancy, sheer helplessness renders any disturbing physical or emotional experience potentially overwhelming; moreover the infant's capacity to communicate or even to understand the nature of such a threat by its analysis in language, is virtually non-existent: at this time therefore repression must be constantly occurring.

It is perhaps just the success of this wholesale repression, together with the steadily increasing capacity for intellectual integration and the development of more complicated patterns of behaviour and capacity for communication with other people, which brings about the change from the explosiveness of infancy to the apparent tranquillity of early childhood. During this latter period repression will still be needed from time to time, but less frequently, as the increased ability of the individual to live in relative harmony with his surroundings makes more of his experience assimilable, and less of it overwhelming and unbearable.

Adolescence combines a vastly increased sexual drive, impelling the individual towards a physical and emotional relationship outside the safe and explored confines of his family, with reactivation of all the earliest personal conflicts and uncertainties within the family, and probably produces the nearest to a neurotic situation which the normal individual will ever experience. For here are some of the essential components of neurosis: the powerful, partly unconscious, instinctual drive, the incomplete emotional integration, and the emergent patterns of behaviour which are not completely successful, but which have roots so deeply anchored in the past, unconscious as well as conscious, that the individual finds it extremely difficult to control or modify them. Nevertheless, the average individual is endowed with an innate capacity to achieve emotional maturity which gives normal adolescence a favourable prognosis, despite the occasionally appalling misgivings of both subject and parent. Certainly there is evidence that the rate, degree, and final extent of emotional maturation, with consequent resilience and stability of personality, owes a great deal to constitution as well as to background and environment.

Abnormalities in psycho-dynamic equilibrium may follow either excessive operation of the mechanism of repression, or its partial or complete failure. Excessive repressive activity can produce powerful disturbances of feeling with complete lack of insight for their origin – phobias, severe mood swings, or obsessive compulsive phenomena; while failure of repression leads to the flooding of consciousness with bizarre or delusional ideas and hallucinatory experiences, which the subject may be unable to distinguish from reality.

Such disturbances of psycho-dynamic equilibrium may be produced primarily by external environmental stress, or by internal biochemical disorder, leading to changes in the mental state experienced subjectively by the patient as symptoms, and observed objectively by the physician in his examination.

Whatever the biological bases of thought disorder, of disturbance of mood, or of alteration of contact with reality, the actual *content* of the disordered thinking, the particular preoccupations and symbolic rituals of obsessive compulsive states, the nature of individual ideas of reference, and the intensely vivid and personal associations of anguish or despair in pathological disturbance of mood, are all directly related to the individual psycho-pathology of the patient, and are drawn from the reserves of unconscious experience.

The homeostatic character of repression was mentioned above. It is one of the characteristics of homeostatic mechanisms in living creatures that they are capable of giving rise to a vicious circle response under certain circumstances. The role of the kidney in hypertension is an example.

Repression is no exception. The influence of complexes, whose emotional charge has been activated while the nature of the relevant experience remains repressed, upon conscious existence is to produce a repetitive experience of anguish and defeat characteristic of neurosis. It remains repetitive, because the greater the anguish becomes, the more rigid is the repressive barrier, and so the patient is prevented from gaining spontaneous insight and thereby achieving the possibility of subjective alteration.

The neuro-physiological basis of repression remains as yet unknown; but its hypothetical existence gains support from the vivid and often highly personal quality of hallucinations and primary delusions, which can be regarded as the direct eruption into consciousness of hitherto unconscious material, when alterations in brain state have led to a suspension or failure of the repressive mechanism. This occurs to a limited extent as a normal accompaniment of sleep, and leads to dreaming. In waking life it may occur as a complication of acute cerebral toxicity or hypoxia, producing delirium; or as an important feature of the major psychoses, in the form of more complex and enduring disturbances of contact with reality.

References and Further Reading

The quotation from J. Z. Young was in *Doubt and certainty in science*, Oxford, 1951.

John Bowlby's classic was *Child care and the growth of love*, Harmondsworth: Penguin, 1953, and his magnum opus *Attachment and loss*, Penguin, 1971.

The Robertsons describe their work, and give further references, in a chapter in *Support, innovation and autonomy*, edited by Robert Gosling, London: Tavistock, 1973. A further thorough review of the subject is *Maternal deprivation reassessed* by M. Rutter, Penguin, 1972.

Another account of the personality is Anthony Storr's *The integrity of the personality*, Penguin, 1963, and of neurosis and the psychodynamic hypothesis, Charles Rycroft's *Anxiety and neurosis*, Penguin, 1968.

Chapter 4

A System of Classification

A convenient and practical classification of psychiatric disorders arises naturally from the developmental approach, from considerations due to the part played by the function of the brain in human behaviour, and from the effects of personal stress in releasing syndromes in reaction to it.

Disorders Attributable to Malfunction of the Brain

These are known as *structural* or *organic psychoses* because the structure, or at least the physical functioning of the cerebral organ, is disordered. They are psychoses because of their disruption of the patient's ability to comprehend, and indeed live in, the world around him. An essential feature is *confusion* of the patient's mental life and behaviour.

The principal headings will be

1 Local disorders of the brain, and
2 Systemic disease affecting the brain as one organ of the body (see Chapter 5).

The category is known to general knowledge among laymen as 'delirium', 'senility', 'softening of the brain', etc.

Disorders Attributable to Severe Mental Illness

These are known as *functional psychoses*. While the brain is undoubtedly abnormal in its function, the illness is not, at present anyway, primarily attributable to cerebral disorder as understood in the above category. Complex interactions of body and stress occur in these conditions, the principal of which are

1 Schizophrenic psychoses – see Chapter 6
2 Severe depression – see Chapter 7
3 Mania – see Chapter 7

This is the group of conditions known to ordinary people as 'mental illness' and 'insanity'.

Disorders Due to Reaction to Stress

This group includes physical and internal stress, but especially emotional experience. They are known as *functional neuroses* or neurotic reactions, the patient retaining in general his relationship with the world.

1 Milder depression – see Chapter 7
2 Anxiety states and phobias – see Chapter 8
3 Hysterical reactions – see Chapter 9
4 Obsessive compulsive reactions – see Chapter 10

These are not separate categories with sharp boundaries, for patients under stress may, and indeed usually do, display and suffer symptoms of more than one reaction at the same time.

The equivalent colloquial expressions include 'worry' and 'bad nerves'.

Disorders of Development of the Personality

1 Mental handicap, in which the intellectual failure is the most evident component, but emotional maturation is inevitably involved (see Chapter 15).
2 Immaturities of personality, essentially emotional in features, and not necessarily involving any intellectual impairment (see Chapter 11).

People around the patient understand the distinction from mental illness and reaction to stress, employing such phrases as 'he's always been like that'.

Further headings are

Psychosomatic Disorders

Discussed in Chapter 13 and

Sexual Disorders

See Chapter 12. These include a variety of conditions some of which could alternatively be described above; for example, functional impotence of recent onset is in effect a neurosis in reaction to stress, or a psychosomatic condition; and constitutional homosexuality is a disorder of development of the personality.

Alcoholism and Drug Abuse

Chapter 14 is devoted to these subjects.

This classification, considered in detail under separate headings, will be found to cover the whole range of clinical psychiatry, with the exception of that special branch of the subject dealing with children. Child psychiatry differs from adult psychiatry in that emotional disturbance in childhood is so frequently expressed in terms of behaviour rather than by any form of directly communicated experience. A situation producing intolerable anxiety in a child may not, in fact, be experienced by that child as a continuing source of fear. Sometimes it will be manifested by a failure of appetite, a disturbance of sleep rhythm, or perhaps by nocturnal enuresis. Habits can betray unbearable unhappiness or fear sometimes more readily than speech. Often, indeed, the child may have neither words for, nor subjective recognition of, the degree of disturbance he displays. Child psychiatry, while resting on the same foundations as general psychiatry, differs from it, therefore, in certain clinical aspects and therapeutic possibilities. In this respect, its relation to its parent subject is comparable to that of paediatrics to general medicine.

Chapter 5

Cerebral Disorder: Acute Confusion, Epilepsy and Chronic Dementia

Introduction

The functioning of the brain is liable to be disordered in any physical illness which affects the whole body or has local effects in the brain itself, so that the student will come across the syndromes described in this chapter wherever he is working in medical practice, whether it be in the patients' homes or in any department of the hospital. Any day he may be presented with mental symptoms and disturbed behaviour in the foreground of a clinical picture, when the important diagnosis lies in the field of underlying, and so far undetected, physical disorder affecting cerebral function.

Delirium (Acute Confusional States)

These can all be regarded as varieties of acute cerebral dysfunction. When this is of recent and reversible form, it retains the same clinical characteristics as chronic dementia, which is the deteriorative outcome of progressive disruption of the structure or function of the brain. But in acute confusional states these characteristics are telescoped together, so that their individual recognition tends to be obscured.

AETIOLOGY

1 Hypoxia and hypercapnia in the brain, with many causes, including carbon monoxide poisoning and lack of oxygen in the air, many handicaps of ventilating power of the respiratory apparatus, lung disease, and circulatory failure of the cardiac output into the internal carotid artery.

2 Anaemia: all the many causes of haemopoietic anaemia (which is, however, usually chronic), haemolytic anaemia and blood loss.
3 Hypoglycaemia
4 Diabetic ketosis
5 Renal failure
6 Hepatic failure
7 Infections, with high fever, and secondary dehydration and hyperventilation
8 Other electrolyte disturbances – dehydration, potassium deficiency, hypo- and hyper-calcaemia, complications of steroid therapy.
9 Cerebral intoxication by poisons (belladonna, industrial and agricultural products, lead, mercury), alcohol, cannabis, or drugs (complications of correct or incorrect doses or mixtures of amphetamine, bromides, barbiturates, paraldehyde, and indeed any drug whose main action is on the nervous system, including general anaesthetics, and many others). Sudden acute withdrawal of these substances may also be an important factor.
10 Nutritional and vitamin disturbances
11 Acute endocrine disturbances in thyroid and other disease, and probably contributing in puerperal psychoses.
12 Acute local and general cerebral oedema and damage, as after head injury and cerebrovascular accidents, or in the presence of cerebral abscess.
13 Epilepsy, which requires a whole section to itself, below.

Very frequently, of course, in very ill patients several of these factors are present at once, giving rise to great difficulty in correct diagnosis, as for example when a drunk man is concussed from head injury, or a patient admitted with high fever also starts suffering from withdrawal in hospital of a customary large dose of barbiturates. This is well illustrated in Case No. 4 below.

CLINICAL FEATURES
The general clinical characteristics include

1 Clouding of consciousness
2 Failure of recent memory
3 Failure of attention, concentration and judgment.
When the cerebral function is impaired, it is inevitable that the

supreme function, consciousness, will be clouded; an impairment on a dimension that leads from normal vigilance, through tiredness to drowsiness and clouding and later to coma. The changes are subtle and complex, and there may be considerable clouding of consciousness without any noticeable drowsiness, and manifest mainly when attention, concentration and judgment are tested. If the brain is not functioning, it is not computing and recording present perceptions, so that when, tomorrow, recent memory is tested, there will be no record, no memory, of today's events. If the failure of recording and recall persists, it gives rise to the typical finding of

4 Disorientation in space and time.

There are further

5 Emotional lability, and

6 Hallucinations, and misinterpretations of external reality, often worse at night.

From these six spring all the rest: delusions and illusions (e.g. that the night nurses in the dimly-lit ward are in fact masked murderers), excitement, panic, disturbance of behaviour, and the entire phenomenon of the frightened and frightening patient who is temporarily out of touch and beyond control.

DIAGNOSIS

Physical examination of the patient may discover the cause or more than one cause of cerebral disorder, and X-ray and laboratory investigations may confirm this. The characteristic syndrome of clouding of consciousness and its concomitants indicates the presence of cerebral dysfunction, and helps to exclude other psychotic states such as acute schizophrenia or severe hysterical behaviour disorders. The most useful single question is 'what is today's date?' The confused patient cannot answer because his brain has not correctly registered the requisite perceptions; the schizophrenic, however withdrawn and bizarre, has access to the basic facts about the world, and if contact with him can be established, it will be discovered that he knows the date, although he may be uninterested and indeed hold strange views about it, as for instance that the world will be coming to an end that day as a result of his actions.

Case No. 4
A retired Irish railwayman, sixty-three, married and with three grown-up children, was transferred from a general medical ward after becoming unmanageably excited, noisy and violent some eight hours after admission for a severe haematemesis. He had a history of intermittent alcoholism which had developed since he had taken over the management of a public house on his retirement from the railway. There were three previous episodes of haematemesis, but this was the first one to be followed by delirium.

On arrival at the psychiatric unit he was confused, noisy, violent, and shouting at the top of his voice 'Murphy's shot me in the bum . . .'. He had in fact received an injection of 10 ml of intramuscular paraldehyde into the left buttock, an hour and a half before his transfer. He settled down rapidly with appropriate treatment in the psychiatric unit, and made an uninterrupted recovery.

Subsequent discussion elicited the fact that several years before, he had had a protracted and rather enjoyable feud with a distant neighbour, which had included an episode when he had gone to make things up over Christmas, had been mistaken by his neighbour for a thief attempting to enter the neighbour's small chicken run, and had been fired at and missed, by the neighbour, with a shotgun.

This illustrates the usual mixture of causative factors. The haematemesis lowered blood pressure and also precipitated hepatic failure. But there were also the effects of withdrawal of regular alcohol, and of a painful and powerful sedative, with escalating fear and excitement in a bewildering hospital.

TREATMENT

Nursing
The first essential is to remember that the patient is frightened, estranged, and for this reason often inaccessible and perhaps frankly hostile to the normal somewhat detached clinical approach.

Nurse the patient in a separate room, preferably with regular and constant attendants who become recognized as friends and protectors, who sit with him when he is frightened, talk to him when he calls out, and soothe him by an understanding presence. Anyone who fulfils these requirements is invaluable; anyone who does not, including special nurses who are untrained or unsympathetic in the handling of this type of crisis, is apt to be worse than useless, unless they rapidly and readily learn. Clearly the room must not be entirely dark, nor need it be brightly lit by night, but moving shadows and dark corners should be avoided. Minimal physical restraint, and no hostility, are the golden rules.

Remove causes
Review existing treatment and the patient's physical state, with the object of ascertaining and treating the underlying cause. This may be any or several of the list already described. Whatever the underlying causes they must be reversed, and such simple measures as the administration of oxygen, securing adequate pulmonary ventilation, hydration and reassuring personal contact are all important.

Large doses of vitamin B and C are administered
There is evidence in some of these states at least that the brain is relatively deprived of them and simultaneously has no access to them in the C.S.F. Usually a series of daily intravenous doses is given.

Sedation
Paraldehyde and barbiturates should be avoided – they have disadvantages and are no longer the best drugs available for this purpose. Diazepam in large doses of 20 mg or more in a flexible schedule, is very calming and a dose at night is helpful. Chlormethiazole (Heminevrin) in doses of 500 mg to 1 g several times daily acts similarly. Chlopromazine and Promazine have long been used to control highly disturbed behaviour, but a safer regime is with Haloperidol in doses of 5–15 mg, by injection, as frequently as required (see also Chapter 16).

The Psychiatry of Epilepsy

The general management and treatment of epilepsy are normally the province of the neurologist, and will not be further considered here. There remain certain important psychiatric aspects of this large clinical problem which demand inclusion:

1 The personal and social repercussions upon the patient
2 The involvement with the personality
3 The involvement with associated psychiatric syndromes
   a) Reactive anxiety or depression
   b) Acute confusion, twilight states and fugues
   c) Paranoid psychosis
   d) Mental handicap, dementia and deterioration

THE PERSONAL AND SOCIAL REPERCUSSIONS ON THE PATIENT

'The worst thing about being an epileptic is not the experience of having the fits; it is the way people are liable to treat you when they find out that you have them.' Here in one sentence, a patient has spoken for all fellow-sufferers. The implications of this are that such patients are naturally liable to react with varying degrees of apprehension, denial and an understandable resentment, to the social predicament to which public knowledge that they are liable to attacks of epilepsy all too often condemns them. The doctor's role here is first to acknowledge and accept this as a fact. In such patients the requirement of treatment includes supportive psychotherapy and active encouragement to enable them to regain confidence in themselves, in other people, and in their basic value to society. It may be necessary for the doctor to intervene to prevent threatened ostracism: explanation to teachers may enable the child to remain in his usual school, discussion with employers may facilitate transfer to a safer post rather than dismissal.

Such personal support is sometimes difficult; but if the doctor concerned with such a patient is neither able nor prepared to tackle it, it is all too probable that nobody else will be. The British Epilepsy Association exists to supplement this kind of need, both for public education and the prevention of avoidable segregation and isolation, but like all such associations for people afflicted with enduring or recurrent disabilities, it must rely upon individual professional support for achieving its maximum effect.

THE INVOLVEMENT WITH THE PERSONALITY

It is possible to encounter two markedly diverse or even openly contradictory views on this subject. On the one hand the consultant neurologist with a practice drawn largely from active and reasonably successful human beings who happen to suffer from epilepsy, and for whom he provides efficient medicinal control, may be inclined to stress that the association between epilepsy and personality disorder is a myth. Dostoyevsky was a lifelong epileptic, wrote most of his novels under circumstances of considerable difficulty and personal privation, and completed what is perhaps his greatest, *The Brothers Karamazov*, after certainly not less than 50 years untreated epilepsy. This is obviously powerful support for the view just expressed.

On the other hand, the medical and nursing staff of those special mental hospitals which used to be called Epileptic Colonies, have often formed a very different conception of the association between epileptic illness and personality. It is from this source that the clinical picture of the epileptic personality tends to be derived: as exemplified by periodic explosive irritability, shallow and facile attachment to philosophical or dogmatic moral beliefs, sometimes called religiosity, and a tendency to decline into a deterioration involving intellectual, emotional and behavioural regression, which suggests, and indeed often denotes, insidious dementia.

The key to this apparent contradiction is to be found in the recognition that epilepsy itself is a symptom complex and not a single pathological entity; and that while this symptom complex can occur against a background of an otherwise fully intact and mature brain and central nervous system, it can also arise as one aspect of an immature, congenitally damaged, or diseased brain and nervous system. Where concurrent developmental failure, structural damage, or disease, are non-existent or negligible, patients with epilepsy will conform to the wide overall pattern of normality in their personality: but where personality disorder is a prominent feature of chronic epilepsy, it is almost certainly the outcome, not of the epilepsy itself, but of the concurrent developmental abnormality, structural damage, or disease, of which the epilepsy is itself simply another manifestation. All that has been said about the management of the predicament of the individual patient in the immediately preceding section applies with equal cogency to personality disorder in association with epilepsy.

INVOLVEMENT WITH ASSOCIATED PSYCHIATRIC SYNDROMES

Reactive anxiety or depression
These have been discussed on page 71 above. They are treated in the usual way, and in the case of severe depression the existence of epilepsy does not exclude the use of E.C.T. if it is otherwise indicated.

Acute confusion, twilight states and fugues
Electrical disturbance impairs cerebral function, so that at the times of the fits, and for varying periods afterwards, associated with anoxia and cerebral exhaustion, the patient is in a confusional state, described earlier in this chapter. Longer-lasting conditions

called *twilight states* occur, in which the patient for hours or exceptionally days, is mildly confused, slow in his movements, and largely oblivious to his surroundings, although he moves around and performs purposive actions in a state of automatism. When this results in a long period of wandering, with the patient later being found, bewildered, far from home and with no memory of what he has been doing, this is called a *fugue*.

Paranoid psychosis

The deterioration of personality mentioned above and below often includes paranoid attitudes and delusions. There is in addition a characteristic syndrome described by Slater and colleagues, in which a full psychosis sometimes closely resembling paranoid schizophrenia occurs, typically after many years of severe epilepsy, the lesion often being in the temporal lobe.

Mental handicap, dementia and deterioration

Epilepsy may occur with and complicate many of the varieties of mental handicap, which is further evidence of the vulnerability of the incompletely equipped or developed brain. In a similar way, epilepsy may develop focally or generally in the course of cerebral cortical impairment in dementia.

Deterioration of the personality after years of epilepsy, mentioned above, is probably a complicated syndrome, with contributions from a worsening of the original cerebral disorder, from anoxic brain damage slowly taking its toll of the cerebral cortex after many periods of cyanosis during the fits, and possibly from intoxication by the unusually large doses of anticonvulsant drugs prescribed in an attempt to control severe epilepsy.

TREATMENT

In all cases this must take account not simply of the epilepsy and its repercussions on the patient's life, but also of specific treatments for the psychiatric syndromes mentioned, removal of treatable causes of mental handicap or dementia, and a review of the effects of anticonvulsant medication prescribed so far, with vigilance for possible effects of over-medication.

Chronic Dementia

DEFINITION

In essence, dementia represents any deterioration of previously normal function secondary to brain damage or disease. It is the chronic syndrome of failure of cerebral function. As the powers of recovery of the brain from damage are poor, many dementias are irreversible, and some physicians reserve the term for conditions in which the deterioration is progressive and the underlying pathology irreversible. The wider usage will be employed here.

INCIDENCE

This is dominated by the age-incidence of senile dementia and cerebrovascular dementia, which are rare below the age of 65, and then increase in frequency rapidly with increasing age, so that one in ten of all people over 65 show some evidence of dementia, and surveys of the very old, over 75, living at home show remarkably high rates.

AETIOLOGY

1 Primary degenerative disease of the brain, especially *senile dementia*, but also a group of idiopathic pre-senile dementias, and the rare Huntington's chorea.
2 Cerebral vascular disease giving rise to *cerebrovascular dementia*.
3 Dementia secondary to other conditions.

Senile Dementia
This is closely associated with the ageing process itself, as illustrated by the steeply rising incidence in great old age. It occurs in both sexes, and is probably partly hereditary, like its converse, longevity. No other cause is known. The essential pathology is the replacement of dead and dying cerebral cortical neurones by neuroglia, with argentophil plaques and neurofibrillary tangles, and the degree of neuropathological change is approximately proportional to the state of advance of the patient's clinical state.

Alzheimer's disease is a form of presenile dementia, with the same pathological changes in the brain, present in severe degree at ages 45 to 65. The cause is unknown; the condition may really represent the youngest cases of the age-distribution of senile dementia.

Pick's disease, with the same age-incidence, appears to be a distinct disorder, with separate neuropathological findings, cerebral deterioration concentrated in the frontal and temporal lobes, and a clinical picture in which the personality is damaged early but parietal lobe features do not appear until later.

Huntington's chorea is a purely hereditary disease, transmitted as a Mendelian dominant. One of the patient's parents must have carried the gene and suffered from the disease if he lived long enough. Onset is typically in middle-age, often when children have already been born, half of whom will pass the disease on to another generation. There is atrophy of the corpus striatum, enlargement of the cerebral ventricles, and diffuse destruction of cortical cells. Clinically, chorea and dementia both appear and both deteriorate over years, reducing the patient to a pitifully degraded state.

Cerebrovascular dementia

This occurs in association with evidence of disease in the brain and elsewhere. The pathology is in the arterial walls with fibrous, fatty and hyaline changes, with small apoplectic cerebral haemorrhages. Only a few cases occur in the fourth and fifth decades, but the condition is not rare by the late fifties, with a rising incidence into old age. There may have been strokes and small cerebro-vascular accidents, and typically the clinical condition is both 'patchy', with some mental functions much better preserved than others, and fluctuating in its downhill course, with spells of rapid deterioration and periods in which the patient holds his own. Symptoms of lability of mood, ready weeping and depression, have always been thought more typical of this form of dementia than the senile variety, and may represent a mild form of the severe emotional loss of control found in the syndrome of pseudo-bulbar palsy after bilateral cerebro-vascular damage.

Dementia secondary to other conditions: this list is of the greatest importance because some of these causes are eminently treatable
a) Brain injury – not only after one accident, but also the 'punch-drunk' syndrome in professional boxers. The possibility of slowly developing subdural haematoma must be borne in mind.

b) Anoxic damage after asphyxia and carbon monoxide poisoning.
c) After infection; many causes but note especially the insidious development of late cerebral neurosyphilis (general paralysis of the insane – G.P.I.).
d) After poisoning, by alcohol, lead and other heavy metals, and other drugs and chemicals.
e) In metabolic and endocrine cerebral disorder; hypothyroidism, vitamin B_{12} and folate deficiency, and the thiamine deficiency of chronic alcoholism are not uncommon. Rarer conditions are Cushing's syndrome, hypoglycaemia, hepatic encephalopathy and hypo- and hyper- parathyroidism.
f) Damage by neoplasm of any type, intra- or extra- cerebral. Meningiomata can grow extremely slowly, with insidiously increasing pressure, and sometimes, in such sites as the falx cerebri or on the olfactory groove, are difficult to diagnose.
g) Normal-pressure communicating hydrocephalus, recognized since 1965 as an easily diagnosed and treatable cause of dementia, often associated with retardation, unsteady gait and incontinence of urine.

CLINICAL FEATURES

The impairment of mental function affects all three aspects of personality: intellect, emotional integration, and behaviour. But in practice the relative degree of evident deterioration in each aspect may vary considerably, producing a variety of clinical pictures. The characteristics of deterioration in each aspect will be briefly described: epilepsy may occasionally be a presenting symptom in any of the varieties of dementia, secondary to the overall cortical damage.

Deterioration of intellect
Failure of recent memory is the most consistent disability. This may be so gross that the patient may be unable to remember the nature or place of his last meal, where he is now living, and the whereabouts or even death of his closest relatives or friends. Questioned on these topics, he may say for example that he has come from home to attend the interview, when in fact he has been living in hospital for several years; that he saw and talked with his wife or his mother that same day, when he may have attended her funeral a few months previously. The tendency to fill in what are in fact

blank spaces in the subjective memory of recent events, by entirely confabulatory accounts for which the patient has no insight whatever, is a characteristic of many cases of dementia.

By contrast remote memory may be relatively unimpaired and may indeed remain for the patient the sole source of vivid interest and recall. Concurrent with the failure of recent memory there is corresponding failure of attention, concentration, and judgment; and with these, a total lack of interest in contemporary events, so that such patients neither read nor discuss items of contemporary news or interest, and are frequently grossly disorientated in time and space.

They are unable to perform simple calculations, to maintain logical thought, to comprehend or interpret abstract ideas or to sustain a normal conversation. Their insight for these various disabilities may be partial, and is then attended by considerable anxiety and unhappiness; but frequently they have no insight and maintain a fatuous and stereotyped social facade, in which impoverishment of thought, narrowing of interest, and extreme shallowness and lability of emotional expression produce an atrophy and obliteration of normal mental life of which they themselves appear mercifully to be unaware.

Typical early cerebral signs are *perseveration* of theme, and mild degrees of *nominal dysphasia*, represented by partial inability to name objects, or paraphasic additional rambling additions to the information requested. These features are very well shown in the following exchange with a 66-year old patient with early cerebrovascular dementia. Shown 10p and 50p coins to add up, she said '4 shillings' (money went decimal five years before this interview: failure of recent memory). When she was then asked to name objects which were given her in succession she answered:

penknife:	'silver sovereign' (perseverating on the theme of money)
safety-pin:	'fourpenny piece' (still perseverating on money and four)
comb:	'a small four-toothed comb' (paraphasic and still stuck on four)
keys:	'a sixpenny bit to come in the door' (dysphasic and still perseverating)

Many neurological syndromes may coexist with dementia, depending on the distribution of the sites of damage in the central nervous system as a whole. An important specific one is *Korsakov's syndrome*, in which failure of recent memory, confabulation and total lack of insight, is combined with peripheral neuropathy. It is usually found in severe chronic alcoholics with secondary thiamine deficiency.

Deterioration of emotional integration
Emotional lability is the most important single characteristic, but as already mentioned, some secondary anxiety or depression may occur. There is also sometimes an associated uneasiness, which may find expression as hypochondriasis or as a querulous, evasive, suspicious hostility. Such patients may be convinced that other people are after their money or their good name. They may then become increasingly isolated, self-concerned, rude, greedy and pitiably lonely. Delusions of poverty, or persecution may make their appearance. In all forms of dementia there may be a characteristic reaction, the *catastrophic reaction*, when the patient is confronted with a task which completely exceeds his abilities, but which would not formerly have overtaxed him. He may suddenly burst into tears, or become childishly or explosively aggressive and destructive, afterwards appearing confused, bewildered and apprehensive. A reaction of this kind in the course of formal intellectual testing is virtually diagnostic of dementia. Owing to the subjective distress which it causes, and because it ruins the rest of the interview, however, it should never be provoked deliberately.

Deterioration of behaviour
This arises naturally as a consequence of the aspects above. But even in the control and display of personal habits, the deterioration may be painfully apparent. Public figures may pick their noses on the platforms of political meetings; shameless and inappropriate behaviour, such as crude sexual advances to casual acquaintances, or masturbation or micturition in public, may be the first sign of something very seriously wrong in a hitherto respected and respectable member of society.

When the patients are still living at home, the principal problems arise when they are alone, and are found wandering lost in neighbouring streets, unable to find their way home; when they start to leave unlit gas-taps open; and when they become incontinent and unable to dress themselves or cook.

Involvement with the personality and with social factors

The remaining resources of the personality try to stave off disintegration and mental chaos. Personality traits, in the early stages, become coarsened and accentuated, and long-controlled and repressed matters may be released. So it is likely to be the pessimistic person who weeps helplessly (dimly aware of his disability, plus a cerebral factor of loss of emotional control), the touchy person has delusions that the neighbours are coming in and stealing his spectacles (he has forgotten where he put them down), and the prim spinster believes that she is sexually interfered with during the night.

The social factors naturally include the support, expectations, and, unfortunately, sometimes the rejection, of society at large, the family, the neighbours, the doctors and nurses, and the staff of the Old People's Home.

Before recognition has led to appropriate care being taken of patients with dementia, they may have slithered into appalling confusion and disintegration in their personal life. Their rooms may be in a state of indescribable squalor and disorder; their underclothes filthy, their belongings jumbled and scattered, suitcases stuffed with rubbish, sweets and half-consumed meals hoarded in cupboards or littering the bed, faeces anywhere. The more sordid and unappetizing their predicament, the more necessary it is to remember the tragedy which it bespeaks. Dementia is a remorseless enemy of the natural dignity of man.

DIAGNOSIS

1 *Clinical grounds*, on the basis of the history and examination described in Chapter 2, and the clinical features recounted above.

2 *Psychological testing of intellectual function by the clinical psychologist.* Intellectual decline from an earlier higher level cannot be proved but can be inferred with confidence when aspects of functioning which are relatively resistant to the deleterious effects of cerebral pathology, such as vocabulary, are found to be measurable at significantly higher levels than recent memory and present cognitive capacity. For example, different groups of subtests in the Wechsler Adult Intelligence Scale are grouped into verbal and non-verbal subscales, so that the overall I.Q. can be analysed in more detail (see Chapter 3).

In confirming the differential diagnosis of dementia from functional disorders, tests for disturbance of learning of complex new material and for impairment of memory are used. The Walton Black Modified Word Learning Test, the Inglis Paired Associate Learning Test and the Graham-Kendall Memory-for-Designs test set the patient standardized problems of the kind described in their titles, and discriminate highly between demented patients and those with no cerebral disorder. Tests in which the patient has to copy complex drawings (the Bender Visual Gestalt Test) are also standardized, but can be adapted for his own uses by the clinician in his interview, just as he may ask the patient to draw a clockface to test him for the jumbling typical of parietal lobe dysfunction.

3 *Investigations of physical disease.* Tests which can yield useful information and cause the patient a minimum of discomfort should be performed first, and when a diagnosis of senile or cerebrovascular dementia appears to be certain, judgment should be used in limiting the number of more drastic investigations.

a) Blood tests. Haemoglobin, E.S.R., electrolytes, including calcium, urea, liver function tests, thyroid function tests, vitamin B_{12} and folate levels, and serological tests for syphilis will detect or exclude many causes.
b) X-rays of chest and skull.
c) Electroencephalography.
d) More advanced neurological investigations may need to be pursued, including lumbar puncture, examination of cerebrospinal fluid, cerebral angiography and air encephalography. The latter shows a characteristic appearance in cases of normal pressure hydrocephalus, with dilated ventricles and failure of the air to pass into the subarachnoid space. The condition of the patient may be made to deteriorate by this investigation, and nowadays isotope encephalography may be recommended instead. The brain-scan allows very detailed screening for cerebral lesions without danger or great discomfort to the patient.
e) Computerised axial tomography with the EMI Scanner is now the most accurate investigation for structural lesions of the brain, and presents no great disturbance to the patient.

The task is to exclude any treatable disease causing the dementia, found in about 15 per cent of cases investigated. Differential diagnosis needs further care in excluding depression, especially in association with Parkinson's disease, when the coexisting slowness and apparent apathy of response makes the distinction very difficult between Parkinson's disease itself, dementia and depression. All forms of depression need consideration as possibilities, with the danger of a withdrawn neglected patient with little to say for himself in interview and concentrating poorly, being regarded as demented, when an eminently treatable condition of depression will be overlooked. Chronic deteriorated schizophrenia also may resemble dementia, as may, superficially, a particular hysterical syndrome known as hysterical pseudodementia or Ganser's syndrome. Here the patient displays a mimicry of true dementia, and answers not only wrongly but too neatly so, being able to answer the classical question 'How many legs has a cow?' with a crisp 'Three'. This may be found in stressful situations, in prisoners in a tight corner, but also with clouding of consciousness in acute confusional states or true dementia.

TREATMENT

Specific measures are applied to treatable causes, and in some conditions, such as hypothyroidism and vitamin B_{12} deficiency, the disability may be entirely reversible, in others, such as G.P.I., usually partially so.

In the case of the non-specific dementias, however, the treatment is essentially palliative, in which after the first essential of acceptance of the patient's disability with kindness, understanding and realism, a variety of ameliorative measures may be tried.

1 Establishment of whatever degree of rapport is possible.
2 Explanation and discussion with the relatives of the implications of the condition and their obligations to the sufferer.
3 Saturation with vitamin B in large doses, as there is evidence of cerebral deficiency in some cases.
4 The drugs claimed to increase cerebral arterial perfusion are probably ineffective.
5 Attention to other conditions: improvement of malnutrition, treatment of depression, relief of cardiac failure, provision of chiropody and walking aids, referral for advice on treatment of failing eyesight and hearing, review of the possibility of relieving incontinence by attention to the prostate or vagina.
6 Prescription of nitrazepam or promazine at night, when confused wandering in the dark frightens the patient or exhausts the relatives.

7 Social and administrative arrangements in liaison with social workers: provision of home-helps and meals on wheels, bath-aids and clean laundry service, visits from community nurses and from volunteers, turning off the gas in favour of safer fuels. Help may be possible for exhausted relatives in the form of day care at a day hospital, or of temporary admission to hospital, and there may need to be further consideration of whether the patient would be better off and safer in a warden-supervised flat, in an Old People's Home or in hospital.

8 The property and affairs of the patient may need to be safe-guarded by referral to the Court of Protection (see Chapter 18).

The aim is to contrive circumstances in which the life of the patient is passed with as little personal unhappiness, embarrassment, or humiliation to others, as is reasonably possible. On these matters the sensible detached but human advice of the doctor should be invaluable.

PROGNOSIS

The prognosis for cases of senile, presenile, or cerebrovascular dementia is a certain downhill course determined by the progression of the illness. Full-time nursing in hospital is needed within a period of some months or a few years, and after admission most of the patients die within two more years. Recognition of this prospect, and management of the case along lines dictated by the necessity for imagination, tolerance and humanity, are the keys to procedure.

References and Further Reading

E. Slater et al.'s study, 'The schizophrenia-like psychoses of epilepsy' is in *British Journal of Psychiatry* 1963, *109*, 95–150. Other classical studies are D. A. Pond, 'Psychiatric aspects of epileptic and brain-damaged children', in *British Medical Journal* 1961, (ii) 1377–82 and 1452–9; and W. A. Lishman, 'The psychiatric sequelae of head injury: a review', in *Psychological Medicine* 1973, *3*, 304–18.

Psychometry for dementia is described by E. Miller, *British Journal of Hospital Medicine* 1975, *14*, 267–70, and 'The clinical assessment of higher cerebral function' by J. C. Meadows in the following pages 273–80. T. Arie, widely respected for developing a fine service, describes 'Dementia in the elderly: management', in

British Medical Journal 1973, *4*, 602–4. There are a number of articles in *Recent developments in psychogeriatrics*, edited by D. W. K. Kay and A. Walk, British journal of psychiatry special Publication No. 6, 1971. For a short book, F. Post's *The clinical psychiatry of late life*, Oxford: Pergamon, 1965, can be unreservedly recommended.

A clear survey of the psychiatric complications of somatic disease – organic, psychotic, neurotic, and deviant illness behaviour – is Z. J. Lipowski 1975, 'Psychiatry of somatic diseases', in *Comprehensive Psychiatry 16*, 105–24.

Chapter 6

Schizophrenic Psychoses

DEFINITION

Schizophrenia is a generic name for a group of disorders characterised by a progressive disintegration of the personality and of its
relationship with the world. Capacity to judge the world fails as
contact is disturbed, and emotional stability and thinking deteriorate, with impairment of personal relationships and of ability to cope.
The name is applied especially to long-lasting states, albeit sometimes relapsing and remitting; transient syndromes of similar
disturbance occurring in the face of apparent stress and improving
rapidly, not to recur, are not called 'schizophrenia'.

AETIOLOGY

Schizophrenia can be regarded as a form of mental illness displayed
by human beings subjected to various forms of stress, the response
being governed by a specific constitutional handicap, not yet fully
understood. The overall situation has remarkable similarities to
studies of diabetes mellitus and grand mal epilepsy. All three
illnesses run strongly in families and much of this increased familial
incidence is certain to be genetic in origin. Specific causes are
found for many cases, leaving a group suffering from the idiopathic
illness in which a genetic predisposition releases the illness pattern,
often but not always, early in life.

INCIDENCE

Schizophrenia has an incidence of about 0·85 per cent in the general
population. Surrounding the clinical concept of the disease itself

is the wider social concept of schizoid personality, estimated to occur in about 3 per cent of the general population. This concept rests on manifestations of social and personal withdrawal, often in association with shyness, reticence, eccentricity and a tendency to suspicion and hyper-sensitivity. A marked combination of the last two traits is not infrequent in otherwise unremarkable characters, and has led to their being described as of paranoid personality.

While it is certainly true that cold, potentially ruthless, dreamy eccentrics, or lonely, diffident, sensitive and suspicious people may often be described as displaying schizoid traits, it is their inability to deal successfully with external reality, and especially intimacy with other people, which links them in practice. This type of personality must be of importance in the aetiology of schizophrenia, for 35–50 per cent of all people who develop the illness previously showed some personality traits of this kind.

High rates of incidence are found in isolated rural areas, and also in the deteriorated parts of great cities. This last finding, and the raised incidence in the lowest social class, is probably largely due to the drift of socially handicapped schizophrenics downhill and into the lonely crowd of the metropolis, although some observer-bias among epidemiologists cannot at present be excluded. Cases of typical schizophrenia occur in all cultures, and in surprisingly similar frequency; they can also be identified from descriptions in the annals of ancient civilisation.

Heredity
Kallmann in 1946 summarised the familial incidence as follows. Starting from an index schizophrenic patient, 10 per cent of the parents will be schizophrenic, 15 per cent of the siblings and 7 per cent of the half siblings. If he marries a normal person 10 per cent of his children can be expected to become schizophrenic, and if he should marry another schizophrenic this figure rises to 53 per cent. Much research has been done on identical twin pairs one of whom becomes schizophrenic, the frequency with which the other twin develops the illness then being found. There are problems with establishing monozygosity of the twins, with allowing for bias caused by finding the twin pair through an illness in the first place, with allowing for possible onset of schizophrenia into future old age, and with the criteria for diagnosing schizophrenia (now known to be very wide in the U.S.A.). As the research has become more sophisticated, the concordance rates reported have fallen,

from a peak of 86 per cent in Kallmann's very large series down to 0 per cent in Tienari's series. The results from identical twins reared apart, a very rare event, have been ambiguous.

Results from adoption studies have started appearing recently, and these should be the crucial test of hereditary factors versus the environment. Children born to schizophrenic mothers but brought up away from them have far higher rates of schizophrenia than do control subjects, proving a hereditary factor in aetiology. Among those carrying out research on the cause of schizophrenia, 'either-or' disputes have become out of date, all now agreeing that there is abundant evidence for interaction between genetic factors and the environment.

No classical Mendelian theory has ever been fitted to the figures satisfactorily: a multifactorial genetic hypothesis is needed. Schizo-phrenics have low fertility, which would be expected to lower the gene pool in the population unless there were counterbalancing high mutation rates or biological advantages to gene carriers who do not develop the illness. The latter is quite likely, and one study reported a high incidence of imaginatively creative people among the grown-up children of schizophrenic mothers, brought up in foster homes.

The contributions to the development of schizophrenia made by schizoid personality (discussed above) and by asthenic physique (probably a minor loading factor) may be mediated partly genetic-ally, although an environmental factor may well be involved at the same time.

Biochemical
Many biochemical theories have been proposed, espoused, tested, and quietly discarded. Progress has been very slow but must continue, for clinical observations constantly point to biochemical possibilities, and the apparent genetic mechanism must be bio-chemical in its mode of operation. Endocrine research, despite precipitation of illness by childbirth and some endocrine distur-bances such as Cushing's syndrome and steroid therapy, has yielded little. Large doses of amphetamine, especially over a long period can lead to a symptomatic schizophrenia indistinguishable from the idiopathic illness, although usually there are present at the same time some features pointing to a toxic psychosis. The same applies to some states caused by heavy alcohol intake.

L.S.D. (lysergic acid diethylamide) in amounts of millionths of a gram will regularly cause great disturbances in the mental state, including severe disorders of the feeling of integrity of the personality, and hallucinations, the whole syndrome bearing some similarity to schizophrenia. At the very least this establishes that minute chemical changes in the brain can cause hallucinatory psychoses, and there are of course many other examples, including mescaline.

Two current hypotheses remain promising. One suggests a disorder of transmethylation, with an accumulation of methylated hallucinogenic substances. This would explain experiments in which administering methionine exacerbates schizophrenia but has no effect on normals, and findings of dimethoxyphenylethylamine, which is closely related to mescaline, in the urine of schizophrenics. A second hypothesis, not necessarily excluding the first, postulates disturbances in central catecholamine synapses. This would explain the psychotic action of amphetamine and the anti-schizophrenic action of the phenothiazine and butyrophenone groups of drugs, which although chemically unrelated to each other both block dopamine receptors in the brain. Kety, the foremost worker in this field, has said that he is more optimistic of better understanding ahead than ever before.

Cerebral
Slater in 1964 reported on the 'schizophrenia-like psychoses of epilepsy'. In a series of epileptic patients with schizophrenia he found that some of the patients, mostly with severe unrelieved epilepsy over many years, and often with the lesion in one temporal lobe, had a typical schizophrenic syndrome, with thought disorder and hallucinations in clear consciousness. They were not a population of usual schizophrenics and the findings point to a cerebral localising factor, perhaps precipitating the illness through perceptual disturbances caused in damaged areas of cerebral cortex. Similarly brain-damage after head injury sometimes precipitates a schizophrenic syndrome.

Family and social theories
In general schizophrenia has been thought of as not being directly caused by personal stress, in the way that neurotic reactions are. Thus incidence rates remained constant in war-time and times of national crisis and are relatively steady around the world. The individual patients' illnesses often have very slow insidious origins, unrelated to obvious crisis. Yet the situation is not so simple.

Careful research counting the numbers of adverse and stressful 'life events' in the lives of schizophrenic patients shows a considerably increased amount of stress in the weeks leading up to onset or relapse, and more subtle problems must be present and uncountable. Social isolation doubtless contributes to the onset of the illness, the patients being caught up in a slow vicious circle in which over decades their schizoid personality robs them of friends, which cuts them off and makes them more eccentric, which in turn makes them less likely to keep in touch with their last acquaintances, and so on into complete withdrawal. In the elderly, partial deafness adds to the isolation of lifetime habits and loss of relatives by death, combined with less flexible perception of reality by the ageing brain.

The clinical observation that the families of young schizophrenics often contain peculiar people with odd styles of communication, has led to theories that patterns of communication in the family are actually causative of schizophrenia. It is claimed that the messages, especially from parent to patient, are 'mystifying' in combining an overt message with a covert one which is contradictory, as when independence is prescribed but hints and actual arrangements seem to sap it and impose protection at home. The patient is said to be in a 'double-bind', which is a deadlocked and 'cannot win' situation with the parent. Different typical patterns in the parental marriages have been identified by different proponents of the theories, one that is well known being the so-called 'schizophrenogenic mother'. The patient may be said to be 'extruded' from the family when he is admitted to hospital, and he is 'scapegoated' by having illness imputed wholly to him, when really the parents are also disturbed people in their personal relationships.

None of these theories satisfactorily excludes the possibility that the parents were disturbed people before the onset of the illness because they were people genetically loaded with schizophrenia, which they then transmitted to the children. Alternatively, living with a schizophrenic child is itself a highly stressful and indeed mystifying experience, and the apparent parental abnormalities may occur after the onset of the illness, and in reaction to it. The varying descriptions of the alleged parental abnormalities do not inspire confidence, and efforts to describe them objectively have not been repeatable. The whole subject has been lucidly reviewed by Hirsch and Leff.

The present state of the evidence is that a family interaction theory as a contributory cause of schizophrenia, although often plausible at first sight in the individual case, is unproven. It must also be remembered that many people develop schizophrenia when they are not living with their parents, and the onset may be in any social circumstances including lonely old age. Multifactorial theories of cause are needed, as in other fields of medicine for many of the major illnesses.

SCHIZOPHRENIA AND ANTI-PSYCHIATRY

Szasz in 1961 in *The myth of mental illness* suggested, using a model of hysteria and extrapolating surreptitiously to mental illness in general, that game theory explained the phenomena best and that there was no actual illness present. Later books allege that awkward people are persecuted by psychiatrists who can never be trusted if they work in the public service, and he takes up an extreme right-wing libertarian point of view in saying that the so-called insane should be subject only to the criminal law when they are in difficulties, and never forced to have medical treatment. The effect is inhumane, in that a disabled uncomprehending and incoherent schizophrenic would have to be left in squalor or danger, while all the psychiatrists are busy practising the only decent form of their work: private practice psychoanalysis with the rich.

Laing, with a background of interest in existentialism, described the world of the schizoid personality sensitively in *The divided self*, 1960, and *The politics of experience*, 1967, and has been influential in shaping views on schizophrenia, especially among those who do not actually meet the seriously ill patients. The account of the bleakness of the inner world is followed by suggestions that schizophrenia is to be understood as a valid form of alienation from the outer world. The symptoms are said to have more meaning than has usually been allowed them, especially in the context of theories of family mystification and if they are interpreted as if they were hints, metaphors, poems or in code. So a schizophrenic brought up by an overwhelming engulfing mother, who never let him think for himself, may say that a witch is putting thoughts directly into his head, this being oblique comment on his situation. Laing is tempted to regard the situation as potentially life-enhancing, and has suggested guidance through the mystical trip into inner space as a form of treatment. Schizophrenics are thought in fact to be innocently sane in their alienation from an insane modern world.

The effect of this theory is not in fact humane: blaming the parents has caused them needless additional suffering on top of the disaster which they have already undergone; the patients very rarely feel that their experiences have been happy – nearly always it is regarded as having been an indescribably horrible nightmare, and many patients never recover enough from this appalling scourge to tell the tale of how they felt.

And Laing has not claimed good results from his treatment.

The impulse behind these views is deeply anti-rational, as stated by a profound critic from outside the medical profession: 'Insanity is represented as a true perception appropriately acted out – society itself is insane, and when this is understood, the apparent aberration of the individual appears as rationality, as liberation from the delusions of the social madness. From individual madness, its heartbreaking pain, isolation, and distraction blithely ignored, is to be derived the principle by which society may recover its lost reason and humanity. The project may be taken as the measure of how desperate is the impulse to impugn and transcend the limitations of rational mind' (Trilling 1972).

SOCIOLOGICAL THEORIES

In social theory those whom the psychiatrists call mentally ill are non-criminal deviants from society's norms. Psychiatrists are employed by the State to label them as mentally ill and to make them conform better as good citizens if possible, teaching them to work again, calling them mad for dropping out of society. The deviance is seen as being amplified by the labelling process, and asylums can be seen as emphasizing the stigmatization of the patient by giving him deprived surroundings and expecting him to be abnormal on all occasions.

The disapproval of diagnosis (labelling) will of course prevent accurate research on schizophrenia from being done. The state of the evidence conflicts with anti-psychiatric and sociological theories, for, as Kety said, if schizophrenia is a myth it is a myth with a very high genetic component. Moreover, it can hardly be a phenomenon of alienation from capitalist society because of its universal occurrence, and because in China 'we think the incidence is the same. But our communities accept the patients more readily and we treat them there. We rely heavily on outpatient services and on phenothiazine drugs, but we do a lot of education of the patient's family and his co-workers so that our patients can be quickly released from the hospital and be accepted by the community' (quoted in Kety, 1975).

CLINICAL FEATURES

The essential features of the illness can be summarised under four main headings, which are however not sharply distinguished from one another:

1 Disorders of thinking, including delusions.
2 Disorders of contact with reality; feelings of passivity and hallucinations.
3 Disorders of emotions.
4 Disorders of movement and behaviour.

The process of thinking itself is disturbed, and the result may include a vague abstractness, in which philosophical terms are used freely but without conveying meaning. The associations of different words may not be clearly distinguished from one another, and logical classification may become impossible. This form of *thought disorder* can be measured by a test of the logical processes used in sorting and re-sorting portrait photographs in rank order of abstract qualities such as 'honesty', in the Bannister and Fransella Grid test.

The feeling that the personality has lost control of body and thoughts and that it is no longer clear where the person ends and the outer world begins (so-called dissolution of the ego-boundary) leads to feelings of *thought-insertion* and *thought-broadcasting*, with feelings that thoughts can be read, that telepathy is occurring, and that the patient is being hypnotised or otherwise mysteriously controlled. Thoughts may seem to be stolen away in mid-train, leading to *thought-blocking*. Ideas of reference are common, with a conviction that everyone is hinting and commenting on the patient's actions and even thoughts. In *primary delusional mood* delusions suddenly occur out of an all-pervading feeling of bewilderment and significance. They may include mysterious convictions of inexplicable changes in the universe or within the patient, affecting him crucially. *Secondary delusions* occur as part of the patient's understandable attempt to make some sort of sense of the ideas of reference and disturbance of thought and feeling

from which he suffers. Such delusions in fact show that his powers
of reasoning and judgement are preserved at least to the extent
that he tries to keep order and system in the world of his experience: delusions are a last desperate stand in the retreat before
mental chaos. But the more ill the patient, the more disintegrated
his personality, the more disordered, unrelated and chaotic are his
delusions likely to be.

The potential impact of such disorder is exemplified by the case
of a young man who, while listening to the radio, suddenly became
aware that the entire programme was about him. This conviction
was absolute, and he found himself waiting for evidence which
would convince another person: he was himself already completely
convinced. During the programme a song 'Don't laugh at me 'cos
I'm a fool' was broadcast. The patient smashed the set. As the
patient's thoughts become more abstruse and complicated, he
may coin new words, neologisms, to express them, and may employ
bizarre compressed turns of phrase. One patient with delusions
of being spied upon by Fascist agents because she was a communist,
said she felt like a 'prawn'. Asked to explain what she meant she
replied that it was like being a pawn, but with an 'R' in it for
Russia. It must be remembered that if she had acted as a prawn
and declined to explain herself in words, her bodily behaviour
would have been regarded as meaningless movements.

Hallucinations are very common, most frequently taking the
form of voices repeating the patient's thoughts, explaining, praising,
criticising, abusing or ridiculing his actions in a running commen-
tary, or even before he acts, thereby often distracting him so much
that no outward action follows; but visual hallucinations including
quasi-mystical experiences are not particularly rare. Sensory
hallucinations are probably responsible for the common delusions
of electrical stimulation, and may lead to the belief that the
patient is being erotically caressed by invisible admirers. Such
experiences may at one and the same time form the subject of
vigorous complaints and obvious satisfaction. This preoccupation
with a vivid but unreal world, of course, releases the patient from
the demands and limits of normal existence, and this withdrawal
from reality underlies almost all the symptoms.

Emotional incongruity is often striking. Apart from his bewilderment the patient may show astoundingly little concern about
the uncanny nightmarish world which he describes as his own.
Ominous revelations, often delivered by hosts of hallucinatory

voices constantly intruding upon his thoughts, manipulations of his body and sensations by electricity, witchcraft or telepathy, and even the constellation of the whole universe brought to bear on his single and defenceless mind, may produce not despair nor even violent alarm so much as querulous irritation or a certain aloof suspiciousness. He may announce some terrible personal disaster with blandness or giggles, maintain he is God while remaining meekly in the mental hospital, or write a matter-of-fact letter: 'Dear Doctor, don't forget I am the main psychological cover for the Queen and it is intended that I should be appointed Equerry to Princess Anne'.

Sometimes mood seems to be shallow, but this may fluctuate with alarming depth and intensity – occasionally persecutory delusions are dangerously acted upon, with murderous attacks.

Ambivalence of feeling may further complicate the picture and play an important part in leading to disturbed impulses or conduct. Most of us are aware that it is part of the normal human emotional response to be capable of both love and hostility towards the same person, although normally such feelings are rarely fully present in consciousness in equal proportions at the same time. In the schizo-phrenic, love and hate, trust and suspicion, joy and sorrow, terror and confidence, may co-exist or alternate so rapidly as to be indistinguishable in the patient's mind. It is not hard to see how such a chaos of mental existence can lead to impulsive action or eminently bizarre and incomprehensible behaviour.

Most of us have encountered conventional descriptions of mad-ness with mythical patients such as the man who believes himself to be a hatstand and remains all day in suitable posture, or the lady who imagines herself to be a teapot and squats with one arm curved like a spout before her and the other hand upon her hip as a handle, constantly asking to be poured out. There are of course no patients as conventionally mad as this, but it is among the chronic deteriorated schizophrenic group that we come most near to seeing pathetic spectacles of this kind. For as their grip upon reality progressively weakens and the content of their minds becomes more primitive, jumbled and chaotic, a few patients may assume and maintain for long periods postures symbolic of some inner stress or experience, just as in the earlier and more acute stages of the illness they may seek to convey to an uncomprehend-ing world otherwise incommunicable feelings and ideas by fantastic gestures, speech and action.

Finally, it is of great diagnostic importance that the schizophrenic mental state takes place in *clear consciousness*, not the confused state of the physically ill patient. He can usually be shown to be orientated correctly, to know the time and place, although his alienation withdraws him from interest in such matters; the confused patient by contrast is disorientated, his perceptual organs and brain not taking in and computing the basic information about the world outside.

CLINICAL VARIETIES

The traditional clinical varieties of schizophrenia are conveniently described under four headings, although the categories are not in fact clear-cut:

1 Simple schizophrenia
2 Hebephrenic schizophrenia
3 Catatonic schizophrenia
4 Paranoid schizophrenia and late-life paraphrenia

The first two can be largely summarised by saying that they differ from each other only in severity and chronicity, and are characterised by early onset, often in the teens or early twenties, a chronic course and all too often an eventual deterioration which may be permanent. In simple schizophrenia the changes are of great slowness, with thought disorder, loss of emotional reactiveness and the appearance of apathetic indifference and ineffectiveness in the real world, gradually increasing in a time span of years, with no acute episodes. Hebephrenic patients more rapidly lose the power of normal thinking and pass into states of emotional fragmentation, bizarre speech, eccentric postures, fleeting hallucinations and disorganised delusions.

Case No. 5
A simple kindly man, who had long been recognised as intellectually unequipped for anything more than the simplest task, had succeeded in earning his living for some years as a bath-chair attendant at a seaside resort. In his spare time he used to attend the local cinemas and other public entertainments in his capacity as a Red Cross worker, of a low but most honourable grade.
He gradually began to develop the conviction that he had within him some kind of mildewed sack, 'like a gall bladder, you know, doctor,

except that it has gone wrong . . .'. This he thought was instilling poison in his system and could only be emptied by his squeezing his sides with his elbows and hands clasped across his abdomen, whereupon the contents of his sack would be driven up the back of his spine to rest above his left ear. He could then release it into the back of his mouth by pulling the lobe of his left ear, and spitting vociferously on to the ground.

The somewhat disturbing rituals were complicated by difficulty in concentration, which proved to be due to thought block, and to vague unsystematised ideas of reference, whereby other people were able to fill his sack with fluid by talking about him. For some years he had made a circuit of the local hospitals, demanding operation for his relief.

He eventually accepted admission to the appropriate mental hospital, where his condition was controlled with phenothiazines and appropriate supportive psychotherapy.

Case No. 6
The twenty-three-year-old daughter of a professional man had just left university, where she had obtained honours in foreign languages, and was preparing to apply for the post of translator and confidential secretary at a branch of the United Nations Organisation. She began to develop doubts about her religious position (her family were sincere but not particularly strict Roman Catholics) and to fear that she might have committed a sin against the Holy Ghost, for which she and the devil were personally and jointly responsible to God. She heard God's voice reprimanding the devil for his part in the affair, and telling him that his last chance of being received back in Heaven had gone.

Evidence of this cosmic battle for her soul began to grow around her. Riding in a motor car with her parents, she saw the car overtaken by blindfolded motor cyclists who shot invisible rays into the car from pistols. (Later she was able to identify this part of her hallucinatory experiences as related to a Cocteau film she had previously seen.) Admitted to hospital at her father's urgent request, through her family doctor, she said she had the obligation of sacrificing herself to save the devil, who was after all only Michael, the fallen Archangel. She refused treatment, pursed up her face and mouth for much of the day, and tried to pull out her own hair. She was eventually persuaded to accept treatment by injection, in the first instance of chlorpromazine, and subsequently E.C.T. She recovered from all her symptoms and was restored to normal health in five months.

The third group, catatonic forms of schizophrenia, include the wild and bizarre postures and activities of the seriously deranged, which may alternate with periods of complete stupor and withdrawal. They may carry the least unfavourable outlook and a single attack may be over in a matter of weeks or months and never recur.

Case No. 7

An attractive young woman of twenty-eight, a spinster and only daughter who had been the chief support of her invalid mother for five years, since her father's death, became gradually more preoccupied, distrait and apprehensive until one morning she was found sitting up in bed staring in front of her, mute and inaccessible. She was eventually removed to hospital where she would stand all day long in a corner of the room staring at the wall. She was incontinent of urine and faeces on occasions, had to be fed, and while permitting herself to be led passively to and from her bed, and to meals, neither spoke nor made any spontaneous movement for weeks on end.

Her eventual recovery was secured transiently in the final instance when a combination of phenothiazine and E.C.T. became available: however six weeks after returning home after a remission, which had interrupted the illness three-and-a-half years from its onset, she relapsed during a quarrel with her mother, walked out of the house, and was found standing up to her waist in a pond about half-a-mile away.

Returned to hospital she made a partial response to a resumption of phenothiazines and E.C.T., and was eventually submitted to open-bimedial leucotomy. This operation produced a brilliant result, in that she recovered completely from all her symptoms, and has since remained well for over six years. Her personality, however, remains abnormal, and she has never married nor expressed an interest in marriage or children; she still believes that she may on occasion have heard birds, bees, and small flowers talking to her.

The fourth group, paranoid schizophrenia, comprises all those disorders with prominent delusions, especially of persecution, often developed into logical systems which could be accepted as reasonable were their premises to be true. The delusions may change little and remain 'encapsulated' without subsequent deterioration of emotions, of integration of the personality or of ability to cope in the world. Syndromes developing in middle life and old age are usually of this type, and are called late paraphrenia, as schizophrenia is so typically an illness with onset in the young.

Case No. 8

A prosperous builder aged forty-four was refused a very substantial overdraft from a local bank against the collateral of his firm and property. This was his first serious business reverse in sixteen years of independent building; and he became morose and disturbed about it.

After some months he suddenly expressed the conviction that people were talking about him because the loan had been refused; and that the basis of its refusal was the fact that the Bank Manager believed that he had syphilis, and had passed it on to his wife and children. He then went about demanding legal action against the Bank Manager, and various other people, and accusing his General Practitioner of having falsified and then published medical reports about him. He was admitted to hospital, having refused to see any doctors, after a suicidal attempt in which he had tried to hang himself; leaving a note saying that no one man could stand up to the devilish and calculated campaign of mind reading, calumny, and persecution to which he had been submitted.

During the course of treatment in hospital he disclosed that his mind was still being read by an electronic machine, in which his thoughts were transcribed into a formula for a new and more terrible atomic bomb. He made a partial remission in response to treatment, and returned to take control of his firm and property; seen for outpatient follow-up and assessment he remains deluded, but can discuss and accept support and re-assurance about his general predicament while remaining a competent builder and manager of his business.

Nearly always however there is an eventual insidious and progressive disorder of thought and feeling, sometimes accompanied by hallucinations, with a splitting and crumbling of existing delusions into diverse and inconsistent fragments so that the final picture is one of decline of the whole personality.

TREATMENT

Supportive psychotherapy
Employed as a technique for establishing contact and gaining rapport with a bewildered, apprehensive or suspicious patient. Formal interpretive psychotherapy has never been found to be a valuable form of treatment, and can be harmfully upsetting.

Admission to a psychiatric unit
Very often required as the only way to defuse and stabilise an escalating situation of fear and mutual misunderstanding between patient and those around him. The need may be urgent, and

sometimes will require implementation of an order under the Mental Health Act to protect the patient without insight into his disorder, or to relieve others at the same time. In mild cases treatment may be successfully instituted at a Day Hospital.

Drug treatment

The phenothiazine group of major tranquillisers has been a major advance in the control of symptoms in acute schizophrenia and in preventing relapse when used as maintenance treatment after recovery. They reduce the level of excitement in disturbed patients, relieving hallucinations, and robbing delusional systems of their tormenting capacity. The effect, the mechanism of which is not known, is relatively specific in schizophrenia, where in large doses, to which schizophrenics are remarkably resistant, the drugs make possible the establishment of rapport and contact with otherwise inaccessible patients.

The parent drug is chlorpromazine (largactil), used commonly in doses up to 300 mg daily but on occasion in amounts three times as great. It can be given orally, intramuscularly or intravenously, important side-effects being drowsiness, hypotension, hypothermia, a rare cholestatic jaundice which is slowly reversible when the drug is stopped, and parkinsonian syndromes and dyskinesias. The latter are relieved when acute by the administration of anti-parkinsonian drugs, although occasional cases of irreversible dyskinesias have been reported in patients treated with large doses over very long periods. Thioridazine (melleril) is used in the same dosage as chlorpromazine but with an upper limit of around 600 mg daily because high doses have been associated with a rare retinal damage. The drug is effective, and has not caused jaundice, but cannot be injected. Trifluoperazine (stelazine) in doses of 5 mg to 50 mg daily is also very effective against schizophrenic symptoms; it causes no problems with blood pressure and jaundice and is useful in promoting alertness rather than drowsiness, but it is potent in inducing the unwanted parkinsonian symptoms.

Unfortunately many patients are reluctant to take medication, and avoid doing so when they are unsupervised. This problem has been transformed for the better by the introduction of depot preparations of anti-schizophrenic drugs, of which the one most employed has been fluphenazine decanoate in oil (modecate). A test dose of 12·5 mg can be followed in a few days by 25 mg, the effectiveness of which lasts for two to four weeks, at which intervals

succeeding doses are given. Another depot preparation is flupen-
thixol decanoate in oil (depixol) in a dose of 20–40 mg every 2–4
weeks. Early results suggest good prevention of relapse and especial
benefit in the more apathetic patient. Pimozide (ORAP) around
6 mg daily, and haloperidol in a wide range of doses, frequently
up to 30 mg daily and on occasion 60 mg daily, are sometimes used.

Although it is not certain that these drugs have improved the
long-term results with schizophrenics ten years after the original
illness, there is no doubt that they transform the situation in the
acute illness, and there is good evidence that in the succeeding
year maintenance medication improves results in the general
run of cases, while possibly not improving the chances that the
very mild cases will remit spontaneously nor curing the severe
and deteriorating patients (Leff and Wing 1971). Follow-up medication should be recommended for several years after the last signs
of active illness.

E.C.T.

(described in the chapter on depression) relieves especially acute
disturbed schizophrenics with severe disturbances of mood, and
rapidly restores contact and normality in catatonic patients, in
whom it may be the most important form of treatment.

The management of chronic schizophrenia in the mental hospital

Many patients are still left with disabilities of personality despite
advances in treatment, and despite modern enthusiasm for discharge and the entirely commendable horror of neglectful institu-
tionalisation, some still cannot appropriately live away from the
care, shelter and protection of understanding staff in an understanding hospital. Further deterioration is preventable when the
hospital is run as an open and encouraging community. Mixing
with people can be encouraged while not being pressed. The sexes
mingle, canteens and social clubs are provided, visitors encouraged
and outside forays promoted. Sheltered forms of employment of
all kinds can be deployed ingeniously to make the most of the
shattered patient's remaining potential, and healing may be further
promoted through art, music, dancing and relaxation classes.

Operant conditioning principles are applied in the *token economy*
to encourage desirable social behaviour such as getting out of bed,
table manners, tidy dressing, learning the Highway code and
coping with time-keeping at a job. Behaviour which is to be

encouraged is rewarded by tokens which must be given promptly and explicitly immediately after the desired response has occurred. Unwanted behaviour is ignored. The environment has to be more strictly controlled than is usual, and the tokens are spent like money by the patient to get privileges which he wants. Very detailed planning and a systematic approach are needed, with close attention to the principles of behaviour modification: in this the participation and indeed leadership of the clinical psychologist will be invaluable. Such a scheme need not be dehumanising; in fact, in many examples it has been used to widen the patients' choice in their lives because they can choose within wide limits how to spend their tokens, and the advance towards independent unstigmatised existence, which can certainly be obtained through the improvement in behaviour resulting from the token economy, is greatly to the patients' benefit.

The management of chronic schizophrenia in the community

The number of schizophrenic inpatients has been falling since 1954, but many have been discharged with some handicaps. Community care has been official policy since the Mental Health Act of 1959, but facilities have often been poor, leading to the poignant questions 'but does the community care?', and 'is it obviously right to transfer care from professionals in the hospitals to amateurs outside?'

Rightly regarded, care in the community involves an organised network of services, deployed imaginatively for the needs of the different patients. Hostels and group homes are needed, for many chronic schizophrenics survive best in a narrow range of social stimulation, being harmed in emotionally intrusive families, but becoming irretrievably lost alone in bed-sitters or in doss-houses. Sheltered workshops provide supervision, satisfaction and the chance of working towards self-sufficiency later, while present slowness and eccentricity are tolerated. Social clubs organised by the psychiatric patients themselves with a less-than-hearty style may help the withdrawn to emerge into relationships.

Families with whom the chronic patients live feel isolated, bewildered and exhausted, frequently complaining that they have been told little of what to expect, less of what to do, and nothing of how to get help when relapse is imminent. High priority needs to be given to supporting these families and educating them about the illness, and in this the social worker has been supplanted in helpfulness by the advent of the community psychiatric nurse. The nurse calling on the family re-assures by his availability and by his understanding of mental illness, and this role is at least as important as his task of supervising the maintenance medication, which is often with regular depot injections.

PROGNOSIS:

Manfred Bleuler's study of 500 cases in 1941 remains the most solid basis for the estimation of prognosis. He estimated that 25 per cent of all cases make a complete recovery from the first attack, while a further 25 per cent show a very marked improvement with slight residual defect. The remaining 50 per cent can again be divided almost equally into 25 per cent who show some improvement, but in whom there is a severe residual degree of disability, and 25 per cent who do not recover at all. Pritchard in 1967, comparing older forms of treatment in mildly ill patients, with regimes including phenothiazine drugs, found that the short-term prognosis had improved but that three years later re-admission rates had not been noticeably improved. Later studies of maintenance treatment in a wider range of cases show further improvement, especially with the depot preparations, as described above.

References and Further Reading

The research on heredity is discussed fully in *The transmission of schizophrenia*, D. Rosenthal and S. S. Kety (eds), Oxford 1968.

Amphetamine psychosis by P. H. Connell, O.U.P. 1958 is a classic study.

A lucid sketch of biochemical theories is by Kety in *American psychiatry: past, present and future*, G. Kriegman *et al.* (ed.) Virginia University Press 1975, where he also quotes the senior psychiatrist in Shanghai.

E. Slater's Study is in *British Journal of Psychiatry* 1963, *109*, 95–150, the work on life events by J. L. T. Birley and G. W. Brown *British Journal of Psychiatry* 1970, *116*, 327–33. The family theories are thoroughly criticised in S. R. Hirsch and J. P. Leff *Abnormalities in the parents of schizophrenics*, O.U.P. 1975.

Lionel Trilling was writing in *Times Literary Supplement* 17 November 1972.

Asylums are anatomised in E. Goffman's book, Anchor Press 1961.

The best trials of drug treatment are J. P. Leff and J. K. Wing, *British Medical Journal* 1971, *3*, 599–604 and G. E. Hogarty *et al.*, *Archives of General Psychiatry* 1973, *28*, 54–64.

For the token economy, see T. G. Tennent and J. R. Marshall, *British Journal of Hospital Medicine*, January 1974, and for the problems of families living with schizophrenia: C. Creer and J. K. Wing in the same journal July 1975, and the excellent booklets from the National Schizophrenia Fellowship.

Schizophrenia by F. Fish 1974 Bristol: John Wright, is a clear systematic monograph.

Chapter 7

Depression and Mania

DEFINITION

Depressive illness is a combination of misery and malaise which occurs either spontaneously or exceeds in duration and intensity the normal reaction to any provocative disaster or misfortune. The misery tends to be compounded of guilt, anguish and despair; and the malaise of exhaustion, insomnia, anorexia, constipation, headache and widespread bodily discomfort.

AETIOLOGY

Many theories of the causes of depression have been put forward, but they need not be mutually exclusive. In fact the opposite is the case, and it is best to consider in all cases a wide spectrum of possible contributory factors adding up and leading to the end-state of depression. In any one case, one factor may be a clear and predominant cause, but several other minor ones may be discernible, as well as others not immediately obvious. This we know from the detailed study of individual patients: an early picture in which the doctor feels that he knows in outline the main causes becomes replaced by a far more complex picture of influences which interact in subtle ways unique for that patient.

Genetic
These conditions, especially those resembling the syndromes described below as endogenous depression and mania, run strongly in families, and a hereditary cause has long been suspected although it is difficult to prove because of the familiar dilemma: the parents who pass on the genes are also the people who bring up and mould the children. It is clear however that a strong hereditary factor

exists but that no simple Mendelian mode of transmission will explain the figures of familial incidence. Either complex adjustments of Mendelian theories are needed if depression is to be a hereditable illness, or, far more plausibly, there is a hereditary loading for vulnerability to the condition, transmitted multifactorially through many genes in the same way as height and intelligence. Whether the condition becomes manifest then depends on the interaction of this heredity with the events of the patient's life.

Physique
It has been suggested, but not satisfactorily proved, that severe depressions are significantly linked with the rotund and obese bodily build, also called 'pyknic'. The association is certainly not a very close one, but if even partially true would accord with folklore which expects the fat man to be jolly but also, in consequence of wearing his heart on his sleeve, to be liable to the profounder melancholy when faced with tragedy.

Sex
These conditions are always found to be much commoner in women than men. This is unlikely to be due to hereditary sex-linkage, as some have thought, and the key is more likely to be found in social factors concerning the lives and roles of women.

Stress
Many forms of stress may precipitate or cause depression, and each person's vulnerability to them will be unique. These reactive factors will be elicited in the patient's history. Bereavement, or other overwhelming personal disaster, material loss, intense disappointment of long cherished hopes, or the threat or certainty of abandonment or betrayal by others in whom the patient has trusted, are examples. The common factor in the personal stresses is the experience of *loss*, but it must be remembered that people suffer in other ways than by the loss of loved ones and tangible objects: one can lose father, mother, spouse, child, and money, but also career, beauty, prospects, virginity, religious faith, self-respect. In the psychodynamic hypothesis, depression is understood as concerning a turning of aggression against the self, especially after the loss of someone with whom the relationship had been tinged with ambivalence between love

and hate. Guilt is then explained as the result of self-reproach for the magical consequences of earlier hateful thoughts ('Although I loved him dearly, sometimes I used to wish he were dead: how terrible to think that that wish might have somehow hastened his death'.) Certainly there is much aggressive tone in the self-reproaches of the depressed, as they savagely accuse themselves of unpardonable crimes and prescribe horrible torments as appropriate punishment.

Research studies of the frequency of bereavement in childhood have shown that this must leave a scar of vulnerability to loss later in life, for the loss of a parent early is found in the history of adult depressed patients with unusual frequency.

The factors causing depression can also occur in wider fields however – a concept of exhaustion and loss of vitality in the whole personality is needed to understand many individual cases, and also the results of social surveys which show for example, that of women with large numbers of young children living in poor accommodation in poor areas of large cities, a high proportion is found to be suffering from depression. Depression may also occur in the course of many debilitating physical illnesses, frequently in the puerperium, and is common as a secondary feature to the stresses of other psychiatric conditions such schizophrenia, anxiety states and alcoholism.

Biochemically the physical final common pathway of depression is probably a complex state of mono-amine deficiency at certain important sites in the central nervous system. This hypothesis when fully developed may explain many suggestive observations, such as the depressive effect of reserpine and methyldopa, the acute antidepressant effect of amphetamines and the longer-term effect of monoamine oxidase inhibitors and tricyclic drugs.

A biochemically established depression has a secondary psychopathological effect on mental life, in the sense that whatever in the patient's past recollection, or present situation, is capable of tragic interpretation, will form a prominent part of his preoccupations. In this sense, depression has been compared to the thalamic syndrome, in which all sensory experience is felt as pain. In depression, all emotional experience is felt as sorrow.

CLINICAL FEATURES

The condition commonly reveals itself in three areas: in *mood*; in the *response of the patient to stimulation*, and in the *functioning of the autonomic nervous system*.

The patient's *mood* is characterized by dejection and unhappiness, with some blunting and withdrawal of interest from the outside world, general retardation of mental and physical activity, indecision, and often subjective difficulty in thinking. Feelings of guilt may be intense and occasionally provide the basis for delusions. Such delusions may be self-punitive, including convictions of impoverishment, or hypochondriacal. For example, the patient may believe that he is financially ruined, or is to suffer some dreadful persecution or disaster; and this belief may then be accompanied by hallucinations taking the form of accusatory voices, which simply din into the patient's ears the same melancholy and appalling ideas with which he is already assailed from the sources of his own introspection. Or he may be tormented by convictions that his bowels are blocked, his brains have rotted away or turned to water, or that his whole body is putrefying and a source of offence to others. The key to understanding these apparently diverse symptoms is the recognition that each is the product of an underlying state of mind characterized by a mood of consistent sadness and abject despair.

The *response of the patient to stimulation* is explicable in terms of the retardation already mentioned. Response to questioning, to the necessity of making decisions, and even to the performance of normal everyday tasks, may become unendurably difficult. The housewife may dread going out to do the shopping, partly because of the physical and intellectual effort which it costs her, and partly because her indecision in the face of various items of choice in the shops makes it almost impossible for her to complete this routine task. The pressure of necessity for examination may then lead to a final breakdown into tears which have hitherto been held back only by a tremendous effort. It is a characteristic of many cases of depression that this effort will have been made, and that a facade of apparent although exceedingly brittle cheerfulness may be the presenting feature of the patient's approach.

Sometimes there is a complicating element of agitation; not only is the patient slowed up but he is also restlessly preoccupied with distressing and painful ruminations. He does not say that he has no thoughts, but rather that he experiences morbid thoughts constantly and fruitlessly going round and round. He may become extremely agitated in the face of quite simple difficulties, and may display what has been described as 'a poorly directed strenuosity, with a certain restless chafing'. There is often a diminished awareness of external events with increasingly painful introspection, and narrowed range of thought. The history reveals how he has neglected his usually beloved garden, never finished decorating the room, given up going out to friends, and initiated no new projects at work. First pleasure in sex and then any interest in it are lost, while laughter becomes a thing of the past.

In the sphere of *autonomic function*, the symptoms of outstanding importance are:

1 Disturbance of sleep rhythm often with early morning waking.
2 Loss of appetite and weight.
3 Constipation and dyspepsia.

The disturbance of bowel function corresponds to the retardation seen in the sphere of thought and action. The bowels are not moved regularly within the usual twenty-four hour cycle, as though the passage of ingested food has become increasingly retarded until eventually the patient is severely constipated. This constipation often bulks largely in the patient's mind, and may provide grounds for some of the hypochondriacal delusions already mentioned. Headache is frequently complained of, but often what the patient is describing proves to be less an ache than a sensation of heaviness, fullness, pressure and fatigue. 'Pressing down feelings' over the scalp may be combined with subjective tenderness and hyperaesthesia. The sensation of a tight band around the head may be regarded as one of the symptomatic meeting-grounds of depression and its ultimately inevitable hysterical overlay.

The pulse is usually slow, the skin warm and dry, by contrast with the clammy sweating skin of the patient with acute anxiety. However, attacks of sweating occasionally occur, often in the early morning, when the patient awakens drenched, wholly unrefreshed, restless and oppressed with morbid thoughts and fears.

During the daytime there is a constant sense of fatigue and listlessness. Everything is an effort and nothing seems worthwhile any more. There is often a marked diurnal rhythm, whereby the most extreme distress of despair is characteristically experienced during the earliest hours. Later in the day the anguish begins, almost imperceptibly, to abate; until by the evening the full horror of the illness is lessened, and, for a time at least, the patient may be encouraged to think it is over. But the next day brings a repetition of the pattern; and while the depression continues to develop, day by day the mood deepens, and the evening relief becomes less certain and less complete.

The patient's *personality* moulds the depression, so that the normally conscientious man is the one who comes to be tormented by savage guilt, the religious loses his faith and feels abandoned by God, and the obsessional ruminates in circles, dithers indecisively and checks trivia more than ever. The hypochondriac is sure that his bowels are blocked and his head feels heavy, while the hysterical personality has a dramatic touch even to her depression. Goya draws Los Caprichos, and Shakespeare writes in Sonnet XXIX:

> 'When, in disgrace with fortune and men's eyes,
> I all alone beweep my outcast state,
> And trouble deaf heaven with my bootless cries,
> And look upon myself and curse my fate,
> Wishing me like to one more rich in hope,
> . . . Yet in these thoughts myself almost despising . . .'

To the patient, all this may seem essentially physical. It may be very hard for him to describe it in convincing terms, or to pin it down to physical symptoms which he can effectively recount. Unable to sleep, to eat, to work efficiently, to hope, or to enjoy any of the simple pleasures of life, he may all too often despair of living; and if his doctor appears to have no understanding of his plight, to die may then seem to him to be all that is left.

Case No. 9
This was a patient who came complaining of inability to think clearly, or perform his normal work, which was that of a designer and producer of cartoon films for a British firm. He was a retired naval officer with an excellent service record, and a successful business career up to the time of the development of the symptoms for which he eventually sought advice. His marriage was not particularly happy, although he had managed to contend with this successfully until a year before. He showed the characteristic symptoms of retardation, failure of judgment, and decision. The picture was completed by his sense of general unworthiness, his conviction of inadequacy and failure, and a feeling

of being below par. All this was accompanied by a disturbance of sleep rhythm with early waking, by loss of appetite, and by lassitude, fatigue and constipation.

The diagnosis was therefore not difficult when the symptoms and signs were elicited.

He responded admirably to treatment, and remained well thereafter. He was in fact responsible for a major full-length cartoon film which won international acclaim. After recovery, and completion of this film, he mentioned at a follow up interview that just prior to his coming for advice and treatment, he had felt convinced that the only possible thing to do was to kill himself.

A further illustrative case in which depression leading to a suicidal attempt was followed by hysterical amnesia, was Case 15, described on page 144.

CLASSIFICATION

Depression appearing apparently spontaneously is often called *endogenous*, implying that external causes have been excluded, leaving internal ones such as physical processes, which are usually manifest in the marked bodily symptoms of the depression. When the depression follows external events which are regarded as having precipitated it, it is called *reactive*. The distinction is, however, unsatisfactory. Whether external events have been sufficiently adverse to account for the depression is a judgment by the doctor imposed on the patient. Depression after bereavement is understandable, but what if no loss has occurred except of a distant relative, or of a dog or a canary? A reactive cause can never be ruled out because one more question to the patient might have revealed the disappointment which looms large enough in his case to trigger the depressive process. The syndromes are not clear-cut and there is a continuum between typical examples of each type: probably all depressions are mixed in origin, resulting from the interaction of factors in the patient's life with his personality and physical constitution, and in mild degree they shade off into normal pessimism.

Simple depression is characterized by retardation rather than agitation, by apathy and inertia, but rarely by delusions or hallucinations. In quality it resembles a normal grief reaction; for example the phase of mourning after bereavement. The depressive phases of *manic-depressive psychosis*, or *recurrent depressions*, are characterized by a greater degree of loss of judgment and of separation from reality; and are more likely to be accompanied by delusions and hallucinations.

Phases of normality, or of mania with elation, may alternate with phases of depression, which are then called *bipolar depressions* in contrast with the *unipolar depressions* in patients who have never so far had an episode of mania. The cycle may vary in duration from days and weeks to months or even years. There may be long intervening periods during which the patient shows no symptoms of any kind, and all combinations of depressive and manic phases are found in the lives of different patients.

Involutional melancholia, a name now used uncommonly, described severe illnesses of the agitated type in late middle and old age. These patients suffer very severely, importunately pace up and down, wring their hands, and often have bizarre delusions of impoverishment and bodily change. Severe adverse moral judgments are passed by the patients on themselves, and they feel damned and a pollution to those around. Severance from reality is most acute in this form of the illness, and therefore, of course, the risk of suicide is correspondingly grave.

Puerperal depression. It is usual for women to undergo a period of emotional disturbance some time within the first ten days of the puerperium, with lability of mood but especially transient depressions with weeping ('the blues'). This may provide the foundation for the development of a depressive psychosis (or mania) in a small percentage, less than 0·5 per cent of women.

These illnesses are usually of relatively short duration and good prognosis. Specific aetiological factors are probably

1 The additional psychological stresses and challenges of pregnancy and labour, with all the emotional significance attaching to the prospects of childbirth and motherhood; and
2 The considerable and sudden biochemical changes secondary to the endocrinological crisis following delivery, in which the level of progesterone in the circulation drops catastrophically with the delivery of the placenta.

Case No. 10
Was a lady in her early fifties who was referred to the Skin Department complaining of infestation by insects. These were imaginary, and she was correctly noted as being hallucinated and deluded during her attendance at the Dermatological clinic. On examination in the Psychia-

tric clinic the presenting features of guilt, self-reproach, agitation and disturbance of sleep, appetite and bowels, with progressive weight loss, gave us the diagnosis. Treatment of her depression resulted in a total abolition of her delusional and hallucinatory symptoms.

Case No. 11
Came on the recommendation of his firm, as an alcoholic. He was a technical engineer in an oil company, responsible for a great deal of difficult and exacting work. He too was in the latter half of life, and had experienced considerable domestic stress, and labour troubles at his job, immediately before the development of his alcoholic tendencies. On examination he was morose, remorseful, wept easily, and confided that he felt unable to tackle his job, and no longer worthy of his employers' confidence. His sleep, appetite, weight and bowels were characteristically affected. Moreover he was agitated, trembling, and had turned to alcohol as the only means available to him to damp down his increasing tension and despair. Again the diagnosis, once made, enabled both treatment and prognosis of a more hopeful kind to be given.

These cases can be multiplied many times. It is important never to overlook the possibility of depression, and to remember the degree of severity which it may attain, with its attendant dangers, in particular the risk of suicide. Brilliant lives have been lost, and untold avoidable suffering has been endured, because these aspects of the problem have been forgotten, or not even imagined. One way of bringing this home is to quote some excerpts from a patient's own letter. It conveys his state of mind, and his impression of his experiences at the hands of doctors whom he had consulted during his depressive illness, but before it was diagnosed. To quote from his letter:

'. . . All I knew – I didn't even recognize it as an illness at all – was that I was getting very tired and finding it difficult to concentrate and to sleep. . . . My dealings with doctors were not very satisfactory. This was partly my own fault since I was in no condition to explain my troubles properly. I was a desperate man in need of help and with no idea how to get it. . . . I first saw my own doctor in the summer. There were various physical symptoms which worried me. Chief of these apart from exhaustion was pain in my heart which had been increasing for the past few months. I was referred to the heart specialist at our local hospital and was told by him not kindly or quietly but openly in the presence of nurses, that I was wasting his time and my doctor's and that I had better forget about my symptoms. He also told me that

I was a bloody neurotic. I went on seeing doctors, trying to find someone who would understand. I think all of them regarded my physical
symptoms as an attempt to evade some issue. Everyone without exception advised me to stick it. They were all wrong. I knew in my heart
I was not fit enough to do so. I wanted to more than anything in the
world, because I like my job which was teaching. But teaching is not
like other jobs. If you cannot do your job the children suffer too. I
was not a malingerer, and I couldn't bear to be thought one . . . .

'If I had had a doctor who I felt really understood my case, and if
I had felt that I would have received sympathetic treatment, I think I
would have gone into a mental hospital then at that point if it had been
suggested. . . . I spent weeks and months wretchedly dragging myself
around, unable to do anything, having lost all hope and not knowing
where to go for help. I thought of faith healers, but I had no faith. . . .
By this time I knew despair. . . . I was too proud and too ashamed and
too tired to be continually hawking myself from doctor to doctor, in
the hope of finding someone who was satisfactory. The one thing that
had hitherto kept me from suicide was the effect it would have on my
mother, who was seventy-eight, and my sister who was thirty-seven.

'I have pondered a lot since over the problem of how some doctors
can be so cruel, thoughtless, and even brutal in some of the things
they say and do. At first one would imagine that the sight of human
suffering would make them more sympathetic. . . . I think perhaps they
are annoyed with themselves because they do not know what to do
about it. A doctor couldn't do his job if he were too sensitive, I suppose.
They have probably only read about people like me in medical textbooks. At best they can only have seen a few cases themselves, and
perhaps they haven't recognized them when they *have* seen them. But
although I criticize doctors I must also criticize and blame myself for
the state I was in. Self-criticism and blame when one is unable to change
is a terrible thing. When it is accompanied by physical debility it becomes
a vicious circle going round and round in utter hopelessness. I often
thought I would be better dead.'

SUICIDE

Death by suicide is a real danger in any case of depression which
exceeds the normal limits of a stable individual's response to
personal unhappiness. In the absence of effective treatment, probably all seriously depressed patients have contemplated suicide,
and at least 20 per cent of them attempt it, of whom about half
are successful.

Suicide rates are higher in men than women. Age rates show a
small peak in adolescence, but then there is a steady rise to the

highest rates in old age. All kinds of social isolation increase the danger. Fortunately the total rate has been falling in this country since 1963: many factors may have contributed to this, including especially safer gas and drugs, but also possibly better treatment of poisoning, and the success of telephone Samaritan services.

Nevertheless, the findings of recent thorough research on a series of 100 suicides are not encouraging. Suicide is actually rare in the mentally and physically healthy, for 93 of the 100 were mentally ill, 70 mainly with depression, 15 with alcoholism, 3 with schizophrenia and 5 with miscellaneous other conditions. Several of the patients were physically ill in addition. Over half were known to have given warnings of possible suicide, two-thirds had visited their family doctor in the past month, and one-quarter were seeing a psychiatrist.

Attempted suicide is many times more frequent than the above, and this is not merely because many more people are saved than die, but because different, but overlapping, groups of people are involved. The rates are rising very rapidly and have become a major cause of admission to medical departments. The bulk of the patients are young, and far more are female than male.

All psychiatric diagnoses are found, but many of the patients are not seriously depressed nor ill in other ways, and a wide variety of motives may be revealed. Most important, naturally, some of these patients desired to die, but were saved. These patients, fortuitously saved from death, will often be severely depressed, as described above. Many, however, make the attempt or the apparent attempt in a setting which shows that the motive is the effect on others: a desperate appeal for help from a position of defeat, an attempt to manipulate people by a method which is becoming common and well-known, or even a bid to get revenge by inspiring guilt in someone who has rejected the patient. Yet other patients appear to have been motivated by a 'gamble with death'. They hazard their lives, and when they survive may feel that this proves they were 'meant to live', this feeling giving encouragement and sometimes acting as a turning-point towards better times.

Assessment of suicidal risk requires inquiry after many factors. The paradigm of a high risk patient can be derived from the above account, and is a depressed lonely old man, who drinks and is physically ill too. Patients should be asked about suicidal temptations, in a gentle series of queries leading from 'does the future look black?', through 'does life seem hardly worth living?', and 'would it be a merciful release to pass away in your sleep and not wake up tomorrow morning?' to direct enquiry for suicidal temptation and even planning. Patients with strongly expressed guilt and self-criticism and those with delusions and hallucinations are in grave danger.

The risk is shown in follow up studies: after attempts at suicide 20 per cent of the patients try again in the following year, and 1 to 2% will die, while the severity or otherwise of an overdose is no reliable guide to the safety of the patient in future.

Attempted suicide is further discussed in Chapter 16.

BEREAVEMENT AND GRIEF

'When a love tie is severed, a reaction, emotional and behavioural, is set in train, which we call grief'. So Murray Parkes opens his book on the subject, an area which has long been neglected by doctors and indeed by others who may be called upon to help the bereaved. Yet grief, he points out, resembles physical injury more than any other mental illness: the loss is a 'blow', the 'wound' gradually heals – unless there are complications. In psychiatric diagnostic terms, there is a reactive depression and symptoms of separation anxiety, and many of the bereaved become ill.

Grief is a process rather than a state, and can be described as a succession of three stages. At first there is a delay or numbness of feeling as the news sinks in, this lasting usually for hours or days, up to a week or two. This is followed by a stage of pining, with waves of yearning for the lost one, and great distress. Reminders may be both avoided and yet sought, and when present increase the distress. In the third stage of depression, the periods of apathy and feelings of futility increase, with preoccupation with thoughts of the deceased. There may be angry outbursts, and sometimes the dead one is felt to be still alive, while often his memory is idealized. In the usual course, the suffering abates after a few weeks, and is becoming very slight some six months later, although occasional flashbacks of yearning may happen for years, as for example on anniversaries. Parkes summarizes the approximate limits of normal grief as being off work no more than a fortnight, no attempts at suicide, no isolation and inaccessibility from friends and relatives, and not having to consult a psychiatrist.

Complications occur, and some people may be repeatedly overwhelmed by yearning and despair for long periods. Guilty thoughts may be involved, distressing the patient further, and lengthening the process of recovery. Children under five years old may appear to inhibit the grief reaction, and in some elderly people, too, there may be no overt affective disturbance, although the opposite tragic situation seems to be common: the utter heart-break of the widowed surviving partner of a long happy and serene marriage. There may be bodily repercussions, with hypochondriacal phobias of disease and death, and certainly increased rate of physical illness and death in the recently widowed. Alcoholics may relapse, and manic-depressives be precipitated into depression or mania.

MANIA

DEFINITION

Just as depression is a combination of misery and malaise, so the opposite side of the coin is an equally pathological combination of elation and energy. It may progress to exhaustion and disaster, so that the patients need treatment and protection.

AETIOLOGY

There is a constitutional disposition to the illness, doubtless largely hereditary. The close connection between mania and depression in the same patient has been noted since antiquity by innumerable writers, and is now codified in the diagnostic category of manic-depressive psychosis, sufferers from which may have repeated illnesses of episodes of either phase of the mood disturbance. Individual relapses may be closely connected with stress in the patients' lives, whether personal, physical, or mixtures of the two, as in the puerperium.

CLINICAL FEATURES

Mild degrees shade off into the normal through a state described as hypomania. By contrast with the depressed, retarded, inert, apathetic patient, a person afflicted with hypomania shows elevation of mood, and an acceleration and extension of stream of thought, with flight of ideas, pressure of talk and apparently inexhaustible energy.

Such patients are restless and excitable, cannot sleep, often will not be bothered with food, and must always be busy, dashing purposelessly about, taking up one activity after another. They may plan or launch innumerable tasks, constantly abandoning one to embark upon another, finishing none, while seeming to thrive upon the mounting chaos of their own contrivance. The content of mental life seems coloured largely by the future, while the past is ignored; the depressed patient by contrast is bogged down in brooding on the past, and feels he has no future. The loss of customary inhibitions shows in sexual flirtatiousness, when the patient must be protected from irreversible consequences of his behaviour, and in lavish over-generosity in spending his money, which may not be recoverable afterwards.

Like depression, elation is an aspect of the normal experience of human beings; and often only gradually and imperceptibly becomes abnormally intense. But when the sense of well-being and confidence not only exceeds all degree of appropriateness to the patient's life, but begins to colour and to cloud judgment and responsibility to a point at which the normal capacity to adjust to reality and manage affairs becomes impaired, then it constitutes a condition of illness, no matter how little the patient may complain of it.

Case No. 12

A young surgeon (thirty-four) in a university town in the Midlands, began to arrange his operating list earlier and earlier in the mornings, and to instruct the Sister in charge of the Out-Patient Department to book more and more cases for him at his Out-Patient Clinic. By the time he was arriving at the operating theatre and expecting to start operating at 5.30 a.m., and had informed the Out-Patient Department that no less than twenty-five cases were to be booked for his afternoon clinics, it became evident that his general judgment was no longer to be trusted. He proved to be sleeping less than three hours a night, to be drinking and spending to excess in his leisure periods, and by the time of his referral for professional advice, which he insisted was quite unnecessary, had begun to delegate both operating sessions and his Out-Patient Clinic to junior colleagues, in order to devote more time to studying investments on the stock exchange, and the probable form of horses in the local races, hoping to raise vast sums of money to improve the general surgical equipment and facilities of the hospital. On examination he was excitable, restless, distractible, and at once arrogantly confident, insistently flippant, and readily exasperated. He had to be admitted to the psychiatric department of an appropriate hospital, where he was with some difficulty persuaded to remain and receive treatment. At the time of his admission, his professional work was in chaos, and his personal debts exceeded £10,000. He made a complete recovery.

In more severe cases physical collapse from lack of sleep and nourishment may follow unless treatment controls the situation. While gaiety and goodwill often form the superficial characteristics of the patient's mood, irritability and exasperation are often near the surface and apt to be provoked by attempts to control or restrain him. Great tact is therefore necessary in handling such patients. In the severe form of the disorder, *mania*, the patient is uncontrollably excited, while the extreme flight of ideas and pressure of thought may render him incoherent. Such patients may violently assault those who endeavour to control them, and in these extreme conditions hallucinations and delusions (often with grandiose content, as of being God or a millionaire) are apt to occur.

But it is not satisfactory simply to regard mania as the mirror-image of depression, as a simple elevation of mood. To the sensitive observer it seems more like an uneasy caricature of bliss, and strange mixed states of mania and depression at the same time are quite common. The nurses may feel embarrassed by tragedy showing through the non-stop jokes, and they watch for the themes from the patient's life which bring him up short and briefly reduce him to tears: 'the words of Mercury are harsh after the songs of Apollo'.

So too, in the psychodynamic hypothesis, the condition is described as a manic defence against depression, a frantic denial of life's tragedy. This was no new insight, being long known to the poets ('If I laugh at any mortal thing, it is that I may not weep' – Byron's Don Juan) and folklore, in the person of the clown who puts on the motley and gives his greatest performance just as his heart is breaking.

TREATMENT OF DEPRESSION

Supportive psychotherapy (see page 258).

Question of admission to hospital
Very severely depressed patients are at risk from death by suicide, and are in any case in need of full-time professional care, so that

they need to be admitted to hospital. Objections based on psychotic features of the depression, as when the patient insists that he is irredeemably damned rather than ill, need to be firmly but kindly overridden, remembering in all cases that depressed patients are indecisive, and any indecision by the doctor will painfully compound this. Indications from the history that past depressions have exhausted the patient or have been dangerous will be noted as requiring further precautions on this occasion. The degree of support, supervision and treatment available outside hospital influences decisions about admission, too: an isolated patient on his own may need to be admitted when another with a supportive family can be treated at home. Many depressed patients are well treated at a Day Hospital, which can also arrange E.C.T. (see below) if necessary. Community psychiatric nurses may be able to help support the family of a patient being treated at home, monitor progress, weigh the patient, administer much of the supportive psychotherapy, and report to the family doctor.

Antidepressant drugs
(i) *Tricyclic antidepressants,* so called because their molecule includes three cyclic groups. Examples are

a)	Imipramine	(Tofranil)
b)	Amitriptyline	(Tryptizol)
c)	Clomipramine	(Anafranil)
d)	Nortriptyline	(Aventyl)
e)	Protriptyline	(Concordin)
f)	Dothiepin	(Prothiaden)
g)	Trimipramine	(Surmontil)
h)	Doxepin	(Sinequan)

Despite claims to the contrary, these different preparations resemble one another in their action and side-effects very closely, and only occasionally does a change from one preparation to another help a patient who cannot tolerate a particular variety. The patients who are helped are typically suffering from the 'endogenous' type of depression, with physical symptoms, more akin to an illness than to normal understandable unhappiness, and there may be a past history or family history of similar conditions having responded to these drugs. With due precautions against possible self-administered overdosage, the drug is prescribed in a small dose at first. The average optimum dose for all these drugs is from 50 to 150 mg in 24 hours, but this is reached gradually over one to two weeks. Much of the daily dose can well be given at night and there is a long-acting sustained-release preparation of amitriptyline (Lentizol) intended for this purpose. First adjustment of the day dose can be achieved by using 10 mg tablets, especially in the frail and elderly, and full doses in the cases of c), e) and g) are usually lower, 60–100 mg.

Side effects are often troublesome, and it is wise to warn the patient that he will be asked to put up with a dry mouth and possible slight drowsiness and difficulty in visual accommodation. Acute retention of urine can occur, especially with large doses in men with prostatic enlargement, and glaucoma is usually a contraindication. There is evidence that extra caution is needed after myocardial damage, as cases have been reported of arrhythmias being induced by these drugs. Depressive illnesses usually start to improve after ten days to two weeks, but a course of ten to twelve weeks may be necessary for maximum benefit. After a satisfactory recovery the dosage should be gradually tapered off over a number of weeks while the doctor checks for relapse. Long-term maintenance regimes are tried in patients who have suffered recurrent illnesses.

The tricyclic antidepressants seem to act by preventing the inactivation and rebinding of the catecholamines, noradrenaline and dopamine, at nerve-endings in the brain.

(ii) *Monoamine Oxidase Inhibitors* (M.A.O.I.) These are thought to act on amine turnover by inhibiting the deamination of the monoamines by the oxidase, so increasing the amount in the receptor sites in the central nervous system. Examples are

a) Phenelzine   (Nardil)   45–90 mg daily
b) Isocarboxazid (Marplan)   10–30 mg daily
c) Tranylcypromine (Parnate)   10–60 mg daily

There is less evidence that these drugs are effective in depression than there is for the tricyclic group, many studies being compatible with the action being that of a mild anti-anxiety drug. Nevertheless a great deal of clinical experience supports an anti-depressant action, and this is often thought to be especially helpful in more 'reactive' depressions and in atypical cases in which phobias and symptoms of anxiety are also prominent. Side-effects experienced by the patients are usually mild and some patients even become dependent on the tablets and reluctant to try tapering them off. The dose is gradually raised from low starting levels over one to three weeks, checking on side-effects, which can include dizziness, dry mouth and an irritable restless fatigue.

A rare important complication is the hypertensive reaction to a combination of M.A.O.I. and certain foods, probably because these foods are rich in amines. A very few of the reactions have been dangerous hypertensive crises usually with severe headaches, and a swing to unduly low blood pressure can also occur. Patients are warned to take a *diet avoiding certain foods*, namely cheese, broad beans, yeast and protein extracts and alcohol. They also should not normally be given general anaesthetics or opiates, adrenaline, ephedrine and amphetamine or barbiturates, and it is a usual precaution not to combine them with tricyclic antidepressants or E.C.T. until the M.A.O.I. has been stopped for 7 days. The patients should carry a standard *card* with these instructions. Non-barbiturate sedatives and chlorpromazine do not give rise to complications.

(iii) L-Tryptophan was predicted on the basis of the mono-amine theory of depression to be a possible drug treatment and is being tried, although there are no widely accepted results as yet.

(iv) Amphetamine and its derivatives transitorily elevate mood and energy in many depressed and apathetic patients, but this is not a lasting treatment of underlying depressive illness, and problems of dependency have turned out to be severe, so that this form of treatment should no longer be prescribed.

(v) Promising new drugs in doses of 50–150 mg are: Viloxazine (Vivalan), Maprotiline (Ludiomil), Mianserin (Bolvidon, Norval) and Nomifensine (Merital). Less is known of their pharmacology.

Electro-convulsive Treatment (E.C.T.)
The modern version of this method of treatment consists in the production of an epileptiform convulsion modified by the specific muscle relaxant drugs such as succinyl choline or suxamethonium under intravenous anaesthesia (often with methohexitone), by the passage of a very small electrical current of the order of 250–500 milliamps, for a duration of up to one second, at a voltage not exceeding 150 volts. The treatment is given with the patient in bed, the first stage being the induction of anaesthesia, which is followed by the intravenous administration of a muscle relaxant, the establishment of artificial respiration with oxygen, and the passage of the current through electrodes placed on the scalp.

For the majority of patients, the application of the current is best given unilaterally over the non-dominant cerebral hemisphere. This produces markedly less immediate post-operative confusion, and is indeed subjectively the most agreeable and the least disturbing technique so far as memory and immediate side-effects are concerned. In the long run unilateral E.C.T. appears to be every bit as effective as bilateral in the vast majority of cases. There may however remain some patients whose degree of agitation and distress, or whose failure to respond reasonably rapidly to unilateral E.C.T. may still make consideration of bilateral E.C.T. advisable. This is a matter for clinical judgment based on indispensable experience.

Whether the treatment is given unilaterally or bilaterally, apart from a temporary alteration in breathing, and a flickering in facial muscles and the peripheral muscles of the forearms, hands and feet, which provides evidence of the adequacy of the dose, there is no physical accompaniment to the patient's response. As soon as the response has been achieved, the gag which is inserted to prevent damage to the teeth or jaws during the actual passage of the current, is removed, an airway is inserted, and oxygen supply maintained until normal breathing is re-established within three or four minutes.

Within five or ten minutes the patient begins to recover consciousness, with no knowledge whatever of the details of the procedure and no memory of anything more unpleasant than the administration of the anaesthetic. After a course of treatments, memory for that period of the patient's life often remains impaired, but it becomes normal again for succeeding periods of time.

Treatment is usually given once or twice a week; the average number of treatments necessary completely to relieve a severe depressive illness is somewhere between six and twelve if it is bilateral, occasionally up to twenty if it is unilateral. Treatment can under special circumstances be given on an outpatient basis, but it is generally preferable to have at least all the facilities of a Day Hospital.

Its general effect is progressively to relieve depression until the patient is restored to full normal health and happiness. This effect is quite remarkable, and the nature of the relief accorded can be spectacular, when a tormented, agitated, weeping, suicidal patient is transformed into a calm, vigorous, active and happy person. Needless to say, psychotherapy before, during and after the course of electrical treatment is part of the whole process. In the early stages its most effective form is essentially that of encouragement and reassurance, based upon an appreciation of the patient's grief and fears. At a later stage, when improvement has begun, the degree to which personal problems may remain to be dealt with will vary among individual patients and will affect the nature of the psychotherapy required. In general, clear diagnosis and fine judgment are needed in prescribing treatment, for just as E.C.T. cannot cure unhappiness itself nor can psychotherapy be sufficient treatment for a severe depressive illness.

We still have an incomplete idea of the way in which this remarkable treatment works, but research into the electrophysiological and biochemical changes accompanying it, in patients who respond, suggests that its effects involve the cerebral cortex, mid-brain, hypothalamus, neural stalk, anterior pituitary and autonomic nervous system; it can further be postulated that the epileptic discharge itself may be merely incidental, a by-product of the stimulation required to trigger off the other and perhaps more directly therapeutic processes. Certainly the spontaneous fits of idiopathic epilepsy seem to produce much less benefit; while the administration of E.C.T. to such patients when depressed is by contrast strikingly beneficial.

Hypnotic drugs and diurnal sedation
The wakeful torment of the depressed patient requires direct relief, using safe and non-addictive medication. Barbiturates now can and should be avoided, because they are highly addictive to some patients, are dangerous when taken in overdose, and need to be restricted in circulation for the social reason of reducing illicit purloining by drug addicts. Sleep can be secured by adjusting the dose of chloral hydrate (1–3 g), dichloralphenazone (Welldorm; 0·6–2·0 g) or nitrazepam (Mogadon; 5–10 mg). Glutethimide (Doriden) and methaqualone (Mandrax) are dangerous in overdose, addictive, and to be avoided. Giving substantial doses of tricyclic antidepressants at night may itself be a measure helping the patient's insomnia.

By day severe agitation may need relief by sedation, and for securing this barbiturates are completely superseded by benzodiazepine tranquillisers such as chlordiazepoxide (Librium) and diazepam (Valium). With the latter, for example, there is no upper limit of dosage, so that one patient may be relieved with 2 mg three times daily, another may require well over 30 mg a day.

Psychosurgery

A number of operations has been developed to cut tracts of cerebral white matter concerned in the pathways in the brain mediating emotional reactions. Thus in the prefrontal leucotomy the principle was the partial isolation of the frontal lobes from connection with the rest of the brain, particularly the thalamus. Neurosurgical techniques have improved the accuracy of this operation, first by undercutting a restricted area only of the orbital cortex, an operation developed by Knight, and then by stereotactically controlled fronto-thalamic tractotomy. The tract appears to be essentially concerned with the emotional quality and elaboration of associations to incoming information. In this sense the fronto-thalamic relationship appears to play a fundamental part in colouring the whole of the patient's personal experience.

Early operations, now obsolete, were sometimes performed in desperation to relieve tormented patients – results were sometimes excellent, sometimes tragically poor; on balance an advance had been made. Now, complications are minimal – there is almost no post-operative epilepsy, and any deterioration of the patients has become almost unknown. Relief, after several months of post-operative rehabilitative efforts, is often brilliant, with many patients recovering completely from being utterly crippled, and being able to leave hospital and cease all medical care. The indications for these operations, now used rarely, are severe unrelieved states of tension, especially in depressive illnesses and in obsessional states, and to a lesser extent in anxiety states. Chronic schizophrenia with unrelievable tension has now become very rare and is not often treated in this way.

Lithium salts – see below under Mania.

PUERPERAL DEPRESSION

This is in general treated as above. Special points are that E.C.T. is especially effective with only a small number of treatments, so that there should be no delay in prescribing it, and that the baby may need especial supervision to protect it from harm if it remains with a psychotically depressed mother. If treatment is at home, family helpers are usually best advised not to take the care of the baby away from the mother, but rather to help her with it.

HELP NEEDED IN GRIEF

An expected death is more easily borne than that which comes like a bolt from the blue, so the medical advisers of the dying can help the relatives by discussing what is to be expected. Practical preparations can then help to lessen the shock, although the extent of what can be done in anticipation of death is limited, not least by superstition. In the first few days of being dazed, the bereaved person needs help with simple decisions and business matters by those close to him, and protection from too much intrusion from friends and neighbours. The funeral, though distressing, is a necessary landmark in working through grief, and is usually afterwards regarded as having been valuable.

Then in the following week people are needed to help run affairs, to be available for comforting, to be neither insistent on mentioning the loss nor falsely hearty in avoiding the subject. The bereaved person has to grieve in his own way at his own rate, needing not 'pity', but company, and words from the heart. Professional help of a more specialized form may be needed to reassure the patient that he is not going mad, to explain that hallucinations of the dead partner are normal, especially at night, to question gently for temptation to suicide, and sometimes to prescribe a few hypnotic tablets. Antidepressant medication is not effective as a routine treatment, but is considered on its own merits, as discussed previously, when normal grief merges into prolonged depressive illness.

Relatives, doctors or clergymen may be able to help in bringing about turning-points in the resumption of outward-looking social life: recommending and prompting, after some weeks or months, a final visit to the cemetery, a holiday with friends, membership of a club.

TREATMENT OF MANIA

Establishment of rapport
This is a prime necessity if any further progress is to be made.

Admission to hospital
It is impossible to treat any form of mania effectively without admission. The patient needs to be protected from exhaustion and from irreversible disastrous consequences of his uninhibited actions,

and this will only be possible in a psychiatric unit with trained nurses and closely monitored medical measures. Sometimes an order is needed under the Mental Health Act to secure treatment for a wildly excited and insightless patient.

Medication with tranquillizers
Chlopromazine, often in doses of 600 mg daily or more, will control the manic behaviour by day, and a large dose at night with or without a hypnotic at the same time, may be needed to secure sleep. Drowsiness as a side-effect need not necessarily be a disadvantage in this condition, but hypotension may occur, and an equally effective regime without these problems is to use haloperidol in sufficient dosage. There is no upper limit, and dosages of up to 60 mg are commonly needed, giving rise to no problems except Parkinsonian side effects.

E.C.T.
In severe mania, a few electrical treatments, commonly three or four within a few days, can be used to bring to an end mercifully an episode of exhausting overactivity barely controlled by large doses of drugs.

Lithium therapy
Salts of lithium, when present in the blood at levels between approximately 0·6 and 1·2 m.eq./litre, greatly reduce the frequency of episodes in patients liable to recurrent attacks of mania, this being well-established in double-blind controlled clinical trials as well as in clinical experience. It is hoped that this effect will be seen also in patients with recurrent depressive illnesses in whom the treatment is being tried. The drug accumulates in the body, rising slowly to therapeutic levels after the treatment is started, so that it is not an effective treatment for the illness in the first few days after admission to hospital. It is best reserved for use as maintenance treatment in patients who have had a second attack of mania and whose lives are therefore in danger of severe disruption from manic-depressive psychosis. Lithium carbonate is usually prescribed, either simply or as a sustained-release preparation, the dose being adjusted in the light of estimations of the blood level, and usually being 800–1200 mg daily. Renal and thyroid function need prior checking and then regular monitoring, the kidneys because the drug is a cumulative one and is excreted in the urine,

the thyroid because of the occasional complication of late goitre and hypothyroidism.

PROGNOSIS

Depressions have a generally good prognosis provided that they are properly diagnosed and treated. Illnesses that forty years ago lasted for months now last the same number of weeks, and recovery will mean restoration to the patient's former health in every way. The problems concern the tendency to relapse, present in perhaps 20 per cent of patients. Of these about 5 per cent undergo a regular series of remissions and relapses, the latter tending to become increasingly resistant to treatment, including E.C.T. A few die by suicide. A small number should be referred for the possibility of relief by psychosurgery, even in old age.

The outlook for patients with recurrent mania has improved with the success of lithium treatment, but this is partial and is a complicated and long-term regime, so that the patient with manic-depressive psychosis still has some liability to disruption of his life at intervals by mania or depression.

References and Further Reading

Kraepelin's *Manic-depressive insanity and paranoia* 1921 has unparalleled descriptions – the account of mania is reprinted in the Wyeth collection of classical papers.

Freud's *Mourning and melancholia* gives the origin of the psychodynamic theory. On classification, read R. E. Kendell *The classification of depressive illness*, O.U.P., 1968, but the masterly clinical study is by Aubrey Lewis 1934, 'Melancholia', in *Journal of Mental Science 80*, 277–340, reprinted in *Inquiries in psychiatry* 1967: Routledge and Kegan Paul, and 'States of Depression: their Clinical and Aetiological Differentiation', in *British Medical Journal* 1938, *2*, 875–8, reprinted in the Wyeth collection of papers.

On suicide, the original classic is E. Durkheim's *Le suicide* 1895, English translation 1957, Glencoe Free Press: the modern classic is E. Stengel's *Suicide and attempted suicide* Revised Edition 1969, Harmondsworth: Penguin, and the up-to-date survey is 'A hundred cases of suicide: clinical aspects', B. Barraclough, J. Burch, B. Nelson and P. Sainsbury in *British Journal of Psychiatry* 1974, 125, 355–73, and reprinted in the Wyeth collection of papers.

Murray Parkes' *Bereavement* Harmondsworth: Penguin 1975 is beautifully written and covers far more than has been touched upon here.

Treatment: the MRC Trial, in *British Medical Journal* 1965, *1*, 881–6, has been much discussed. Its design was not perfect, and it certainly illustrates the great difficulties in getting agreed results in this field. Further reading: 'Differential effect of unilateral and bilateral E.C.T.', J. J. Fleminger et al., in *American Journal of Psychiatry* 1970, *127*, 430–6; 'The practical management of lithium treatment', M. Schou et al., in *British Journal of Hospital Medicine* 1971, *6*, 53–60, reprinted in *Contemporary psychiatry* T. Silverstone and B. Barraclough (eds), British journal of psychiatry special publications; 'The work of a psychosurgical unit', P. K. Bridges and J. R. Bartlett, in *Postgraduate Medical Journal* 1973, *49*, 855–9.

'The words of Mercury are harsh after the songs of Apollo' is the last line of *Love's Labour's Lost*.

Chapter 8

Anxiety States and Phobias

DEFINITION

A state of continual irrational anxiety and apprehension, sometimes flaring up into acute fear amounting to panic, accompanied
by symptoms of autonomic and endocrine disturbance; with
secondary effects on such other mental functions as concentration,
attention, memory, and judgment.

AETIOLOGY

Anxiety states are the commonest mode of presentation of
psychiatric disorders, and make up a considerable proportion of
the complaints which bring patients to their general practitioner
or to the general out-patient departments of hospitals.

The feeling of danger, and of fear of what might happen,
reported by the patients points to the best way of understanding
what anxiety is: it is the person in a state of alarm and prepared-
ness for dealing with dangers that beset him. In animals the
reaction of the organism to physical danger is itself a preparation
for survival of the danger, for fight or flight. In humans the
danger may be social rather than physical, confrontation with
an angry father rather than with a hungry tiger, so that anxiety is
the *specifically human danger signal.* It is therefore in moderate
degree an adaptive response, without which we could not pick our
way through the hazards and difficulties of life, but capable of
being exaggerated, severe, and harmful in some circumstances,
requiring medical relief. All human beings are capable of developing this reaction if the threat to their confidence and well-being
is sufficiently severe.

1 *Heredity* doubtless contributes to individual differences in liability to anxiety states.

2 *Anxiety as a learnt response.* Children learn to be anxious in situations which they experience as threatening. Upbringing by insecure parents who themselves experience the world as a series of terrifying threats will endow the children indelibly with numerous and irrational fears, and contribute to the development of a dependent immature personality. These fears may certainly be passed on unintentionally, as when a mother is terrified of thunderstorms but is keen to bring up her children without this fear. Her intended reassurance 'there is nothing to be frightened of' during the storm cannot calm the toddler who senses the sweating, trembling and panic, and therefore knows and learns that there *is* something to be frightened of. Single terrifying experiences in childhood sometimes crystallize into lasting phobias in adult life, the origins of which the patient cannot remember. One of Freud's patients had a fear of masks, and Freud eventually reconstructed that this must have originated when, as a child, the patient had been taken to see his recently-dead mother laid-out ready for burial. The patient could not remember this, but inquiries in the family confirmed that this had indeed happened.

Many anxious responses to physical and social dangers are of course deliberately and systematically taught by parents to children as part of training for independent life. For our own safety we need to be frightened by a fire, a car approaching at speed, or by a man in a raincoat who invites us into his car, on our way home from school. We further learn to feel anxious in extremely subtle social situations, when in danger of breaching rules and codes of acceptable or desirable behaviour. If the anxious response then becomes excessive, the patient may come with a complaint of a symptom that he blushes when wanting to talk to a girl, is tongue-tied with his boss, sweats and panics in examinations, or trembles when eating in public in a restaurant. After an experience of acute severe anxiety, a *panic*, the patient may become stuck in a pattern of irreversible retreat. He avoids crowded shops because the prospect of another panic there is unbearable. Then he may avoid any shops because the panic *could* recur in any enclosed space. Never daring to test himself again, he is confined within barriers of confidence which, without help, he cannot surmount. At a time of further stress and insecurity, he feels frightened even to leave his house lest panic recur in the street, and before long he may be housebound. Specific fears of situations which must therefore be avoided, such as the fear of going out or the fear of masks, are described as *phobias*, and so-called phobic states can be regarded as a variety of anxiety states in general.

3 *In the psychodynamic hypothesis* anxiety has figured as an internal danger signal, the threat being that dangerous repressed thoughts and desires might be pressing to return to conscious life and cause disaster. Anxiety is found when there is *conflict*, but the conflict may itself be unconscious and unknown to the patient, sometimes concerning the reawakening of deeply buried material from as long ago as infancy. Nevertheless, conflict at a conscious level is readily identifiable in many anxious patients, and may concern, for example, duty or loyalty conflicting with pleasure or the line of least resistance, in friendship, marriage, sex, parenthood, career or other concerns. No doubt conscious immediate anxiety is reinforced from unconscious sources by repressed reservoirs of fear related to past experience.

The specific fear complained of may point to more hidden factors, either by *symbolism* or through the doctor's imaginative study of the whole context. A phobia of snakes – serpents – may symbolize the threat of succumbing to sexual temptation as in the story of Eve, and any phobia may be found to involve hysterical mechanisms.

4 *A secondary hysterical component* may determine to some extent the nature of the symptoms, for example the specific phobias encountered, and their effect on the patient's life and the lives of those closely connected with him. Then the incapacitating symptoms themselves serve motives unrecognized by the patient, but influencing or manipulating the environment in ways otherwise impossible of recognition or achievement. The neglected wife, who becomes eventually bedridden by an intense phobic anxiety about being left alone in the house, or going out alone to do the shopping, and who therefore finally secures the undivided although reluctant attention of her husband, provides an example.

CLINICAL PICTURE

Anxiety itself may dominate the patient's subjective mental state; or, alternatively, the patient may complain of physical symptoms which are the outcome of the normal adrenergic component of anxiety, such as tachyardia, restlessness, loss of appetite, insomnia, sweating, tremulousness and loss of weight. Periodic episodes of acute fear amounting to panic are common.

Some patients may experience either their basic anxiety, or these crises of blind and overwhelming fear, accompanied by physical sensations of choking or suffocation, or a feeling of impending collapse, mainly or exclusively in response to certain specific stimuli. For example they may be unable to face travelling on an underground train or going in a lift, or they may be acutely afraid of venturing out alone on the one hand, or meeting people or going into a crowded place on the other. In practice phobias restricted to a single type of experience are rare, and what usually happens is that the underlying and persistent anxiety is heightened to an unbearable degree by the activation of the particular phobia concerned. *Agoraphobia* so called, the fear of going out into spaces away from home, is typically such a complex syndrome, with other fears and phobias being present, and often a life-long history of tension, anxiety, fears and dependency in personal relationships, in the face of stresses which are seen as threatening.

Physical symptoms include the autonomic accompaniments of anxiety already mentioned, which in turn lead to the vegetative disturbances, weight loss, exhaustion and insomnia. The patients complain of tension, and they mean this literally – the skeletal muscles are in fact tense when they should be relaxed.

Headache, and of a characteristic kind, is a common symptom. Its cardinal feature is its painful quality, by comparison with the sensations of fullness, heaviness, bursting, compression or passive tenderness of the scalp, more often encountered in depressive states (see page 107). The headache in states of anxiety and tension is frequently described as throbbing, stabbing, burning or 'raging' in quality; its distribution is usually parieto-occipital, or 'behind the eye'. In its most severe form it has many of the characteristics of migraine, with which it may anyway blend in some cases.

Sleep disturbance takes a characteristic form, the patient being unable to get to sleep for hours, tossing and turning restlessly, and finally falling into a broken slumber often disturbed by vivid and terrifying dreams from which he may awake tense, sweating and trembling. It is common for patients to claim that they have had less than an hour of unbroken sleep for many weeks or months.

Hypochondriacal preoccupations are common, and may be related either to the physiological symptoms of anxiety on the one hand, or to the apprehension and sense of impending disaster on the other. The patient may scrutinize his own bodily sensations vigilantly, ever-alert for the tell-tale change which signals the presence of the dreaded cancer, brain tumour or late effects of venereal disease.

The syndrome can be brought home to the reader if he recall the state of himself or his friends at a very anxious moment, say on the morning of the wedding day, or just before entering the room for a very important interview or crucial professional examination. Before the examination, he feels tense, on edge, sweaty, and has little appetite for food at breakfast, after a restless night's sleep. He checks his pens several times, although he knows for certain that he has enough with him, and fear mounts within him as the tube train stops in the tunnel, threatening him with being trapped and eventually late. Outside the examination hall, friends are restlessly pacing up and down. Diarrhoea and frequency of micturition attest to autonomic disturbances. Some people waiting have blotchy red patches on neck and face; many smoke more than their custom, using the effect of nicotine on the autonomic nervous system. All the systems of the body are affected in anxiety, and this also includes sexual function, for, as described later (page 176) fear makes men impotent and women frigid. These feelings, multiplied many-fold, are those complained of by the anxious patients.

Case No. 13
A twenty-year-old medical student was certain that he had developed pulmonary tuberculosis. He based this upon his perpetual lassitude, occasional night sweats, and a difficulty in concentrating upon his reading, keeping up with his case work in the wards, and enjoying either his studies or his leisure as he had been wont to do. His appetite had failed, and he was losing weight.

On examination he was tremulous, tense and sweaty, but his erythrocyte sedimentation rate was eight, and his chest X-ray normal. Discussion revealed a number of anxieties related to his parents, girl friend, his digs, and his forthcoming examinations. The aetiology, diagnosis and treatment in this case were decidedly similar to that of Case 2 already quoted on page 39.

Case No. 14
Mrs J.H., a housewife of twenty-six with a son of four and a baby daughter of eighteen months, had begun to suspect that her husband might be becoming interested in one of the girls at his work. He was coming home late, was occasionally absent for hours at a time over

weekends ostensibly to pick up a little extra money by odd jobs, and displayed less tenderness to her during the past eighteen months than she had grown to expect. She developed symptoms of general anxiety and tension, which rapidly focused themselves upon an inability to go more than a few hundred yards from her house without becoming faint and fearing that she might fall down unconscious in the street.

Eventually she reached the stage at which she could no longer take the children out, do the shopping, or care for the house. Neighbours did what they could to help, and her husband was undecided about what line to take with her. One morning she began to feel panic-stricken, and feared she might drop dead in the house. She got a neighbour to ring her husband's place of employment, and to call the doctor. He returned precipitately from work to find her in bed, with a very high pulse rate, gasping for breath, and convinced that she was soon to die. Her distress led to her doctor's arranging for her admission to hospital, where she settled down; and whence, after six weeks in the psychiatric department and a considerable exploration and revision of the marital situation between husband and wife, she was able to return home and resume a normal existence.

TREATMENT

An essential first step in the management of the patient is the exclusion of physical diseases mimicking an anxiety state. The common condition to be excluded is hyperthyroidism, which is found at all ages but typically in young women, and which may present with tension, restlessness, tremor, sweating and loss of weight, and which is in any case often found to be associated with true anxiety in the same patient. A rare mimicking condition is recurrent hypoglycaemia and a very rare one, phaeochromocytoma.

A principle to be borne in mind when embarking upon the treatment of anxiety, is implicit in the account, given above, of the reaction as a danger signal. Flashing red lights sometimes function wrongly, and then, after the most careful investigation of the situation, it is sometimes correct to switch them off and proceed further, but this is the exception. Danger signals are not to be switched off heedlessly; rather they demand removal or mitigation of the danger, so that the warning signal, in the natural course of things can then abate.

1 *Psychotherapy*. This is the treatment of choice in every case and corresponds to a process of exposing the source of the threat and defusing it as a source of danger to the patient. Simple supportive and explanatory measures may alone bring enormous relief,

but sometimes interpretive psychotherapy, brief or prolonged, or group. or family therapy will be indicated because of the setting in which the anxiety occurs in a particular patient. These forms of treatment are described fully in Chapter 19.

2 *Psychological Methods of Relieving Physical Symptoms.* *Relaxation*, whether induced with or without hypnosis (described on page 282) counteracts the bodily feelings of tension, and the patient, feeling better and reassured, becomes more calm and confident. These states of calmness and confidence in turn reduce the autonomic overactivity, with resulting further improvement in relaxation, abatement of tachycardia and cessation of sweating. The patient learns an effective safe technique, with no disadvantageous side-effects, and can help his treatment along by his own efforts at home as well as in professional sessions.

Biofeedback techniques can be regarded as a highly sophisticated development of this kind of treatment. A machine monitors a physiological measurement such as pulse rate or blood pressure, and the patient is given the findings as feedback at the time. If, by such techniques as relaxation, he can change an abnormal measurement towards normal, he is made aware of the result straightaway, and can rapidly develop more effective techniques. The method is still being evaluated.

3. *Drug Treatment.* a) Minor tranquillizers such as Chlordiazepoxide (Librium), Diazepam (Valium) and Lorazepam (Ativan) relieve the symptoms of anxiety very effectively, acting partly centrally in the brain and partly by reducing the activity of spinal reflex centres. With Diazepam there are tablets of 2 mg, 5 mg, and 10 mg size available, and flexible regimes can be used, using the smallest doses compatible with substantial relief of symptoms. The important side effects are drowsiness and the corresponding danger when driving, and the tendency to habituation and to take gradually increasing dosage in long-continued anxiety states. The drugs are very safe in the case of poisoning by overdosage.

The main clinical disadvantage of these drugs lies in the way that the excellent relief they afford from the symptoms may stultify wider considerations in treating the whole patient. He may regard the tablets as the only treatment he requires, and once they are started may be reluctant to cooperate in the often hard work of psychotherapy directed at the underlying problems.

b) Mono-amine oxidase inhibitor drugs, described fully in the chapter on depression, are sometimes useful in states with symptoms both of anxiety and depression.

c) Tri-cyclic antidepressant drugs are sometimes helpful in treating secondary late depressive features.

d) Beta-blocking agents. The physical accompaniments of an anxiety state are due to beta-adrenergic stimulation. Specific receptor antagonists may therefore be used to block the stimulation. Propranolol (Inderal) in a daily dose of 30–80 mg may prevent palpitation and tremor, and may be combined with minor tranquillizers. Caution is needed in the presence of cardio-vascular disease.

e) Barbiturates, formerly used for mild sedation by day, sometimes for interviews under intravenous sedation, and occasionally for continuous sleep treatment, are now best replaced for all these purposes by Diazepam and similar drugs.

f) Nocturnal sedation is often needed. It is effective and safe with Nitrazepam (Mogadon) 5–10 mg, although even this safe drug should not be started lightly. One doctor can easily start prescribing it, but at some time in the future the patient and perhaps another doctor will have the problem of stopping taking it and resuming normal sleep.

4 *Behaviour Therapy: techniques for treating phobias.* Clinical psychologists inspired and developed these techniques, which are now widely used. Only loosely based on learning theory, they consist of empirically developed methods of unlearning the phobias and retraining the patient in desired forms of behaviour.

In *desensitization by reciprocal inhibition*, the aim is to desensitize the patient to the feared object of a specific phobia, by gradually associating it with relaxation, which is the converse of anxiety. The patient lists his feared situations in order of severity and enters them very gradually, starting with very mildly frightening ones, while being relaxed, for example under light hypnosis or with drug sedation. If he has a phobia of thunderstorms, the feared situation would be represented by a tape-recording of thunder, which in each session, as the patient lies relaxed, is played a little more loudly. Eventually the patient is relaxed, not anxious, in the presence of loud thunder. Some treatment proceeds well using the patient's imagination to conjure up vivid scenes of the feared situation, in other cases the principal measure is real-life testing, for example by means of going for walks of progressively increasing distance, at first with and then without the therapist, to treat agoraphobia.

In *implosive therapy or flooding* the procedure is very different.

The aim is to expose the patient fully to his feared situation, and to prevent him from fleeing from it. Normally he avoids the situation and thus damps down his anxiety but never actually conquers it, whereas in this form of treatment he is forced to be 'flooded' with anxiety. If the phobia is of cats, he is kept in the room with the therapist and a cat, despite being made severely anxious by this situation, and he is not allowed to escape. Discussion with the therapist then emphasizes that the patient has faced the worst and survived it, so that never again need he, nor will he, be terrified of being near a cat. Further sessions are needed, to emphasize the result and allow for more discussion, but usually the treatment succeeds rapidly with single phobias and is much less time-consuming than desensitization.

In *modelling* the therapist again uses encouragement, persuading the patient to follow his model behaviour as he first goes near, then touches, a small kitten, then a large cat. All the while the therapist is available to discuss fears, encourage progress, discourage retreat and confirm good results.

Behaviour therapists have tended to modify their methods with experience, finding increasingly that they get better results when, in addition to meticulous attention to the techniques of retraining, they succeed in building a good rapport with the patient, and allowing him to discuss wider aspects of his problems. There is in fact a much less clear distinction between behaviour therapy and psychotherapy than formerly: they are fortunately tending to combine in a general attention to the patient's anxieties by means of personal and psychological methods.

5 *Day Hospitals* are often very suitable places for the treatment of severe anxiety states – much treatment can be arranged in a short period, and relaxation classes and practice walks for agoraphobic patients can be organized, as well as individual or group psychotherapy.

6 *Self-help*: Agoraphobics Anonymous has helped many patients by telephone contact, newsletters, etc.

PROGNOSIS

The outlook for the promptly treated acute anxiety state is good, and intervention must be authoritative to bring it to an end, for the untreated or unsuccessfully treated one is likely to become increasingly complicated by secondary depressive and hysterical features with the passage of time. Agoraphobia sometimes becomes intractable in this way, with the family inextricably involved, and the limited routine becomes the only foreseeable way of life of a limited person.

Patients with life-long anxiety-prone personalities improve considerably with reliably available support at times of stress. Truly specific single phobias are rare, but are often curable.

References and Further Reading

The authoritative monograph is I. M. Marks 1969, *Fears and phobias*, London: Heinemann. The whole subject is discussed psychodynamically in C. Rycroft 1970, *Anxiety and neurosis*, Harmondsworth: Penguin. See also M. H. Lader, 'Psychophysiology of clinical anxiety', in *British Journal of Hospital Medicine* 1969, 2, 1448–51, reprinted in *Contemporary Psychiatry* T. Silverstone and B. Barraclough (eds), British journal of psychiatry special publication 1975; and V. Meyer and E. S. Chesser 1970, *Behaviour therapy in clinical psychiatry*, Harmondsworth: Penguin (see also p. 290).

Chapter 9

Hysterical Reactions

DEFINITION

Hysterical reactions represent the attempt, never fully conscious and frequently totally unconscious on the part of the patient, to obtain relief from otherwise intolerable stress, by the exhibition and experience of symptoms of illness.

This is our definition. But two earlier definitions will be quoted, to bring out an important distinction, all too often misunderstood by the student. The two earlier definitions, both of them admirable in their way, can be seen to contribute to the misconception which it is one of the objects of this section to correct. These two definitions are:

(1) Hysterical symptoms are symptoms not of organic origin, which are produced and maintained by motives never fully conscious, directed toward some real or fancied gain.
(2) Hysterical illnesses represent the attempt, never fully conscious and frequently completely unconscious on the part of the patient, to obtain some advantage from the exhibition and experience of symptoms of illness.

Note the emphasis in both of the above definitions upon *advantage*, and *real or fancied gain*. The implication of this is sometimes taken to be that hysteria is a deliberately purposeful reaction and that the discovery of the advantage to which it is directed, is necessary to both its understanding and diagnosis. This can even go so far as to lead a student to say 'this can't be hysteria; because I can't see what the patient is getting out of it . . .'. In fact the truth is that hysterical reactions do produce relative advantage and relative gain, in the sense that the *relief* from otherwise intolerable stress, postulated in the definition which heads this section, does represent for the patient a less disastrous or totally hopeless or unendurable predicament than that which preceded the hysterical reaction, and which has been mitigated by it. But nevertheless it is rare for a patient with a hysterical reaction to be actually better off as a result of it, by comparison with the situation which prevailed *before* the stress, which provoked the reaction, had occurred.

AETIOLOGY AND PSYCHOPATHOLOGY

Stress may be *emotional stress* or conflict, arising from the life situation of the patient, and different for each patient. But it is important to realize that the stress may be represented by *physical illness*, its pain, disability and uncertainty. When the physical illness affects the brain, as in dementia and other neurological conditions, this itself directly affects the patient's overall resilience and equilibrium. The stress may also be represented by serious *mental illness*, especially depression or schizophrenia.

This situation, in which a serious physical or mental illness is accompanied by additional hysterical symptoms, not caused by organic structural pathology, is the notorious so-called *hysterical overlay*, a source of ignorant and unjustified hostility to the patients. There is also a dangerous trap for doctors here – if the hysterical symptoms in the foreground lead to a hasty conclusion that the patient is 'hysterical', then thorough physical and psychiatric examination may be neglected, and the correct diagnosis of the underlying condition can be missed, with disastrous consequences for the patient.

Other factors interact with stress in bringing out the hysterical reaction, in particular there must be an *illness-rewarding situation*, of which there are many varieties, both specific and general. In the army and in prison, reporting to the doctor and being certified sick ensures relief from parades, or admission to the less harsh regime of the sick-bay. Hysteria tends to be frequent in these institutions, with the presence of stress and of illness-rewarding situations, so the authorities arrange disincentives and make it difficult to get access to the doctor. At university, examinations are stressful, and if doctors' certificates retrospectively attesting to illness on the day of the examination, were capable of securing good degrees, no doubt there would be a high incidence of hysteri-

cal illnesses. The authorities take steps to make *aegrotat* degrees
hard to obtain and low in status.

A familiar situation in which hysteria is encouraged by rewards
is *compensation neurosis*. This term is loosely applied to patients
whose disability has followed accident or injury for which
compensation is claimed and either disputed or not finally
settled in amount. There is frequently physical damage as a result
of the accident, but long after this has healed, symptoms, identical
with those experienced by the patient during the earlier stages of
disability, persist, and may even become more severe. These are
often accompanied by anxiety, but in some cases may be regarded
by the patient with surprising equanimity. This latter acceptance
of hysterical symptoms, sometimes amounting to complacency,
was regarded by Janet as characteristic, and has since been known
as *belle indifférence*.

*The underlying mechanism in such cases is usually a sincere
conflict in the mind of the patient which he is unable to solve*; its
basis is the desire to resume work and accept recovery on the
one hand, which is opposed by grave misgivings on the other hand
as to whether he will really be as fit as he was before the accident,
and whether, if he resumes work and finds he is not as fit, he will
be able to re-establish a valid claim to sympathy, consideration, or
further financial compensation for his sufferings.

Such cases are exceedingly difficult to treat, since so much
depends upon the patient's confidence not simply in his physician,
or the fairness or generosity of those responsible for compensation,
but ultimately in himself, and it is the underlying failure of confidence in himself which all too often produces and maintains the
hysterical disability. In this it is aided by the powerful financial
disincentive to recovery: proof of permanent illness equals money,
whereas evidence of recovery and return to work equals no money,
because the employer rebuts the claim. There may be further
conscious or unconscious motives, for example resentful retaliation
against the authorities; and the strength of the patient's proud
commitment to the struggle and determination to win the case,
can be very great.

Nevertheless, the actual position of the patient is often far less
satisfactory than if he were able to accept recovery, and as the
case grinds on he will be examined and counter-examined, kept
upon the rack of uncertainty about his future, while his chances of
ultimate recovery after years of illness become smaller and smaller.

Chronic anxiety states, severe depression and even the precipitation of previously marginal or undiagnosed schizophrenia, may complicate the situation. In all cases it is clear that complete final lump sum payment to end the unsettled prospects and possibilities of litigation is absolutely essential, and urgently needed with the shortest possible delay, before treatment directed to the symptoms is likely to succeed. It is often then found that after final settlement treatment is easy and the symptoms improve remarkably easily and rapidly.

Hospitals, by definition places where the ill are looked after kindly, afford asylum from stress through illness, so that hysterical illnesses are liable to abound in all departments. They are also always frequent among patients consulting their family doctor. Hysteria mimics and is parasitic upon physical illness, and where the later abides, there will the former be found also.

But the main reward from illness is a very general one, stemming simply from the other people affected by the illness, especially the patient's immediate family. *The sick have a role*, with many rights and privileges. They must be looked after, be excused work, and be paid while remaining at home. A patient who is known to be sick necessarily affects someone, somewhere, who will be moved to help him.

Personality factors and individual differences in the patient's circumstances further affect the liability to develop a hysterical illness under stress and in the presence of an illness-rewarding situation. *Hysterical personality* is one such loading factor, in which the insecure person tends to respond to the stress of rivalry, responsibility and the emotional demands of adult life by submissive reactions and the appealing helplessness of illness. Children frequently develop hysterical illnesses, and so do the mentally handicapped. In fact among these may still sometimes be found the crude and bizarre syndromes, the blindness, the paraplegia, the extraordinary gait, formerly found in the hysterical illnesses of the population at large when it was less sophisticated. Consultation rates for psychosomatic symptoms are high among immigrants and their illnesses comprise many hysterical disorders.

These groups of people and the situations which they are in when especially prone to hysterical illnesses have common factors of significance. In the first place, they are people in positions of weakness. Grown men may be able to get their own way straightforwardly, but children must wheedle, immigrants fend for themselves on the edge of society and hysterical personalities manipulate through the emotions. And in a society dominated by men, 'women conquer by swift and strange surrenders' (Oscar Wilde). One way of acquiring influence in a position of weakness is from the sickbed.

The other common factor is a relative lack of facility with words. Immigrants are at a disadvantage in trying to communicate in a language not their own, but can point to their abdomen, make noises and encourage the doctor to examine them. Backward peoples and children excel in acting, dancing and rituals which may be of a sophistication well ahead of their verbal skills. The mentally handicapped will be especially handicapped in the complexities of language. In dementia, fluency with language is lost early with the onset of forms of dysphasia. The hysterical personality may be perfectly articulate, but typically is adept at communication without words, in the language of the eyes and the body, by hints, drama, tears and flirtation.

Hysterical illnesses, we can now see, are communications, by the weak or weakened, in the language of illness.

The *mechanism* of symptom production rests upon the normal capacity of human beings to form concepts with an emotional significance and imaginative elaboration, and to react to these concepts as if they were real. Hysterical symptoms appear to be produced by a dissociation of normal mental processes, whereby certain concepts, patterns of activity and related associations are separated from conscious awareness and relegated to the unconscious area of mental life. Here the effects of suggestion cannot be counteracted by insight or criticism, and the patient's capacity to comprehend or modify the experience is correspondingly limited.

Malingering: In the most superficial types of hysterical illness the advantage tends to be comparatively obvious to the dispassionate observer, while the symptoms directed towards it may be equally transparent. It may indeed be difficult to draw a line between deliberate and conscious malingering on the one hand and the more superficial type of hysterical illness on the other. Nevertheless, true malingering is rare, if only because of the capacity inherent in every human being to believe what seems to be necessary or desirable to him; this in itself is an effect of suggestion and may explain why hysteria, in contrast to malingering, is comparatively common.

CLINICAL FEATURES

The simplest forms of hysterical reaction involve the loss or distortion of normal motor or sensory function. Blindness, deafness, anaesthesia or paraesthesia, paralysis or disturbance of reflex motor activity, for example in vomiting, may occur. Symptoms may be psychological rather than primarily physical: loss or disturbance of consciousness or of memory (amnesia), hysterical hallucinations, or disturbances of behaviour may also occur.

Reasons for choice of symptom

a) *The patient's knowledge of disease* will be a crucial factor: one cannot mimic the unknown. This accounts for the naivety of the crude syndromes of the unintelligent, and the notorious complexity, difficulty and subtlety of hysterical conditions in doctors and nurses.

b) *Existing and familiar physical illness* – the patient brought up by a mother liable to migraine develops hysterical headaches; the epileptic has additional hysterical convulsions; the patient with multiple sclerosis suffers symptoms of hysterical overlay not accounted for by the lesions in his nervous system.

c) *Social trends* are involved in determining which illnesses are commonly mimicked. Gross anaesthesias, blindness and deafness are now rare hysterical syndromes; what are commonly seen are headache requiring extensive investigation to find organic causes, backache the cause of which remains elusive, compensation neurosis as already described, and a mimicking of severe depressive illness in patients distressed by appalling housing conditions and hoping for a letter from the doctor pressing for rehousing on medical grounds.

d) *The patient's own concept of the illness* as it emerges will affect the picture. This may involve *body-language* and *symbolism*, in so far as the symptoms may produce some partial solution to the patient's difficulties with relief of subjective anguish, and may symbolize the sort of solution which would be emotionally acceptable to him, although in practice it may not be possible. An example was a very self-controlled bank manager who after months of severe, personal stress suddenly broke down into a condition of mutism, with in addition weakness and shaking of the right arm. These were found to be of hysterical type, and he was later able to say that their onset was at a crisis when he was in danger of betraying his dearest principles by nearly striking and swearing at his own son (who was the instance of the stress). The hysterical symptoms prevented him from striking or speaking, and symbolized his powerlessness and speechlessness in the face of his problems. They also secured him help by means of the sickness-role and treatment in the psychiatric unit. Another example is Case No. 16 below.

In summary therefore, hysterical illnesses occur when a patient under stress, in an illness-rewarding situation and with unique personal factors of his own, develops symptoms mimicking physical illness, which ensure that he is treated as ill. This provides some relief from the stress, although often only temporarily and unsatisfactorily. In flight from stress he may jump from the frying-pan into the fire.

Clinical examples
Some examples from clinical practice will both illustrate the features just described, and link them to some of the aetiological factors already outlined.

a) *Hysterical Reaction to the Patient's Life Situation*

Case No. 15
A lady in her late fifties, in a state of considerable distress, was brought late at night to the Casualty Department of a large hospital. Her clothes were wringing wet up to her waist, and her handbag which had been found near her was empty. She had been discovered crawling along the ground on the banks of a nearby river.

On examination, apart from mild shock and exposure, she did not appear to be suffering from physical illness; but she was totally unable to remember who she was, where she had lived, or indeed any details of her personal life whatsoever. Nevertheless she knew that she had been brought to hospital, she knew the meaning of the uniforms of the police who had brought her, the nature of the ambulance service, and such everyday items of information as the use of a telephone, telephone directory, and so forth. She was admitted as an emergency, and the following day with little difficulty, by a simple technique of encouragement and free association, the following story emerged.

She had been widowed eighteen months. Her husband, to whom she had been devoted, had been an engaging but somewhat irresponsible commercial artist, who had died prematurely and in debt, and she had had to sell their house, which was mortgaged, in order to meet his obligations. She had no surviving relatives of her own and had obtained part-time work as a seamstress in lodgings to maintain her independence and self-respect. During the preceding winter she had become ill with pneumonia, and on discharge from hospital had had to change her lodgings. She had subsequently become exceedingly depressed, and to her great shame had made a suicidal attempt, taking some aspirin tables and attempting to cut her wrists. This had earned her a second hospital admission, and eviction from her second lodgings. Immediately prior to the incident which led to her admission to this hospital, she had sought out her husband's only known relatives with the intention of asking them if they could help her. However, although she had received a superficial welcome from them, they had not inquired and she had not been able to summon the determination to tell them of her present predicament, or indeed to imply how desperate had been her plight since her husband had died. She had bought a small bottle of gin and some more aspirin tablets and had gone to the river presumably with the intention of drowning herself when sufficiently fuddled to make this possible. But after the purchase of the gin and the tablets, she could remember nothing more. Circumstances suggested that she must have begun to wade into the river, but found the whole thing beyond her, and had developed an hysterical amnesia as the last psychophysiological defence against total helplessness, hopelessness and despair.

With appropriate supportive, individual and rehabilitatory measures, she made a complete recovery, and remained well under follow-up supervision thereafter.

Case No. 16
A young woman of twenty-two was referred to Outpatients with a six-year history of total incapacity from continuous generalized shaking and trembling movements, which resembled myoclonic jerkings. Extensive and exhaustive investigations at a number of previous hospitals had effectively excluded structural damage or disease. The history of the complaint was that she had begun to fall helpless to the ground, and to lie there twitching, when she was sixteen, shortly after her parents had refused to allow her to continue for a further year at school, since she was required to earn money for the family; while at about the same time their own chronic and severe marital disharmony had become increasingly apparent to her and to the rest of the family. Within a year her attacks of falling had been followed by increasing periods of disability due to the jerking, twitching and trembling movements, until after two years she had become totally helpless and disabled.

On examination the generalized twitching, jerking and trembling of all her limbs, head, and body, effectively prevented her from reading, writing, feeding herself, or indeed looking after herself in any way whatever. She was helpless and bedridden, and her sole recreation was listening to the radio.

Careful and intensive individual psychotherapy over a period of only two months revealed a considerable reservoir of repressed resentment and despair at her own relationship with her parents, and their relationship with each other. Numerous incidents were recounted, after which she was momentarily relieved of some of her tension. Finally, after a brief period of continuous sleep, she was enabled during recovery to begin to move her limbs regularly and under control, and within two weeks of emerging from continuous sleep was completely restored to normal health and control of movement. Discussing the entire illness in retrospect she said spontaneously: '*I just couldn't stand up to* the continual fighting and quarrelling at that stage in my life. . . .'

b) *Hysterical Reaction following Head Injury*

Case No. 17

A married woman of fifty-four complained that following a car accident three years before, she had lost all sensation in the tips of her fingers, heard music as 'a painful noise', found her eyes blurring and her head aching whenever she attempted to read for more than a few minutes.

She and her husband had been passengers in a neighbour's car at the time of the accident, when the car had skidded, mounted the kerb, and hit a wall. She had suffered slight concussion, was not unconscious for more than one or two minutes; and had at no time displayed signs of neurological disorder on clinical examination. Neither compensation nor any kind of litigation following the accident were involved or contemplated.

In her previous history she had always been a timid anxious person, and had been complaining of symptoms of flushing and exhaustion, associated with the menopause, at the time of the accident. There was also a complicated family situation arising out of the fact that her eldest daughter had been deserted by her husband, had divorced him, and was now contemplating a second marriage to the son of the driver of the car in which the patient had been riding at the time of the accident. The patient herself had been anxious about this second marriage, and after her accident it was postponed by mutual consent between the families, pending her recovery.

In view of the length of the history, and the chronicity of the symptoms, she was admitted to hospital for a complete overhaul and treatment, and was in fact cared for in the psychiatric unit.

An important aspect of her investigation included systematic psychological examination. This showed a characteristic impairment in critical thinking, and in her capacity to make use of the functions of concept formation, integration, and comparison, which would have been appropriate to her general level of intelligence.

Nevertheless, with careful specific individual psychological treatment, and general attention to emotional problems which had complicated the aftermath of the accident, she began to recover confidence; only for a time to display a marked secondary depression, with guilt about the effect of her illness upon her daughter's life. This in turn yielded to appropriate antidepressant medication (see page 118) and continuance of individual psychotherapy. Eventually she made a complete recovery within three months.

In this case a subtle but important disturbance of mental function had been connected on the one hand with physical damage, in no other way detectable, secondary to mild concussion, and on the other hand with the emergence of patterns of hysterical reaction for which it was partly responsible, but which were in no other way referrable to the physical damage. This particular type of syndrome is seen sufficiently often after head injury to be worth noting; and its relationship both to the head injury and to personal psycho-dynamic factors, will often enable it to receive satisfactory treatment, if sufficient attention is given to the problem.

c) *Hysterical Reaction following Injury to Other Parts of the Body*

Case No. 18
A married man of thirty-four was crippled by total paralysis and anaesthesia of the right arm, of seven years' duration. He had in fact married during the course of this disability, and his nuptial celebrations had been one of the few human endeavours not significantly impaired by his incapacity. The marriage was happy, and his wife went out to work to supplement his sickness benefit and relatively meagre interim compensation payments (see below).

The symptoms had developed very soon after an alarming accident at work, when a service lift in which he was placing trays from a canteen where he worked as a general waiter, began to descend prematurely while his head, arms, and upper part of trunk were still inside it. He at once cried out, and attempted to free himself; but his right hand had become caught around the handle of the trays and his right arm was dragged down with the descending lift until his right shoulder became jammed between the top of the lift cabinet and the lower edge of the opening to the lift shaft. At this point the lift was stopped and he was rescued.

He was then found to be shocked but not seriously injured. His right shoulder was bruised, and the overlying skin showed superficial abrasions, as did his axilla. He could move his fingers, arm and shoulder, but the fingers were stiff and painful, his neck ached on the right side and he had been not unnaturally very considerably frightened.

The paralysis and anaesthesia were first observed seven days later, during which interval his arm had been immobilised on a raised aeroplane-type splint in front of him, while X-rays and electro-myographic investigations into the possibility of joint or nerve damage, were being undertaken at a nearby hospital. Total paralysis and anaesthesia coincided with the removal of the splint following the hospital's verdict that no serious damage had been done.

On examination, seven years later, his total flaccid paralysis and anaesthesia extended from the finger tips to the tip of the acromion on the right side: secondary trophic changes in the skin of the palm and flexural surfaces of the fingers were apparent but not complained of; nor did the distribution of motor or sensory loss correspond to brachial plexus or spinal root or chordal patterns. Nevertheless his arm was useless, senseless, and oedematous, and he reported that he had already been advised to consider assenting to its amputation as a flail limb. This was confirmed from his notes.

A case for compensation against the owners of the restaurant concerned had been in varying degrees of complexity and completion with an interim weekly payment to the man of roughly one-third of what he had been previously receiving as wages. Following admission to hospital, effective and final settlement of the compensation claim was made a matter of agreed priority. It was achieved by a long overdue compromise; in the form of a lump sum paid to him irrespective of his further recovery or disability. Thereafter – and for the first time – effective treatment became possible: and in response to it his case followed much the same course as that of the girl with the multiple shakings and tremblings described on page 145. His eventual recovery after three and a half months was complete and total; and seen for follow-up at yearly intervals, he has remained well and able not only to resume employment, but to use his right arm and hand for fine work, particularly in his spare time hobby as an electrician and repairer of radio and television sets.

Case No. 19

A married man of forty-eight years fell twenty-eight feet when a ladder on which he was working, cleaning lamps in a railway terminus, over-balanced and crashed to the platform. This ladder should have been steadied by the permanent exertions of his mate, who had in fact been temporarily absent procuring them both a cup of tea from a nearby canteen.

The man's immediate injuries included fracture of the pelvis, of three ribs, and considerable shock. His fractures had united and his general condition had returned ostensibly to normal after three months in hospital, but in fact he continued to complain of extreme weakness, shakiness, and an inability to set foot on a ladder. He also had multiple pains in his pelvis and dorso-lumbar region, and was being urged by a firm of solicitors to press a claim for compensation against the railway authority, or alternatively against the firm of contractors for whom he was working, as a lamp-cleaner and servicer at the time of the accident.

Once again attention to the medico-legal situation was clearly essential as a first step. Careful and penetrating inquiry elicited the fact that neither the patient's union, nor his wife and family, were in favour of his pressing the claim, since they both recognized that in the long run it would almost certainly have to be preferred not against the railway authority, nor against his firm of contractors, but against his mate; who had been absent from his post at the bottom of the ladder. The ladder itself had been subsequently examined and found to be in no way defective.

When the solicitors who had been advising him were obliged to recognize this, and had been able in the light of it, to satisfy themselves that neither the railway authority nor the contractors would be liable for damage, the claim was dropped. Within six weeks, the man's morale had begun to improve and he made a final recovery from his disability with purely out-patient supportive treatment. His own comment on the situation, when promised and finally provided with the clarification which it had clearly required was: 'Thank heaven I know at last where I stand. . . . Now I think I can begin to get better and go back to work with an easy mind'.

The underlying conclusion which inexorably emerges from all these considerations is that hysterical symptoms are never unimportant: often because of their crudity and transparency to everyone but the patient, they provoke contempt and hostility, but always they are a warning that a human being in distress has found no better solution than a partial surrender. To unmask them is easy. To restore to true health the patient displaying them is often exacting and difficult, but there can truly be no doubt about which way the doctor's duty lies.

TREATMENT AND PROGNOSIS

Careful exclusion of physical illness or other mental illness underlying the symptoms
While it is a serious mistake to miss physical illness or severe depression, harm can also be done by repeated investigations, especially in an atmosphere of uncertainty. After many consultations and X-rays the patient may become committed to his illness

and there is always the risk of a borderline or doubtfully normal finding to frighten him further. An announcement by a distinguished physician that the cause has been found: sacralization of the fifth lumbar vertebra, osteophytes in the cervical spine, a little spasm in the barium meal pictures, and any subsequent doctor probing for stress caused by personal problems will be greatly handicapped. The wise doctor investigates carefully, once, and then if he has no diagnosis takes more history before ordering more barium studies.

Removal of the underlying and provocative stress
Successful treatment of missed physical illness removes the hysterical overlay. Relief of severe depression by E.C.T. may be just as dramatic as the original 'hysterical' symptoms. If the stress is caused by personal problems, it may or may not be possible to relieve it completely; the measures needed may not be accessible to the patient's doctors, or it may be literally impossible to change a deadlock. Efforts to help require: —

Psychotherapy
This often involves the people and environment around the patient. Supportive or interpretive individual psychotherapy with the patient (described in Chapter 19) embarks upon elucidation of the stress, the conflicts of motivation and incentives known and barely known to the patient, and study of the effect of people around who are appealed to by the illness. Complicated bargaining may be needed, in different combinations of interviews with different people. Hints and compromises are the order of the day.

Anyone involved in the illness-rewarding situation may need to be drawn in. From the psychiatrist's point of view, the family doctor is one of the people to be involved in discussion and negotiation; but conversely, to the G.P. trying to sort out a similar situation, hospital specialists are people whose role is to be studied and allowed for.

With the patient and his family, discussions of motivation and genuineness are to be avoided. The aim is to maximize the advantages of health and minimize the rewards of illness, in so far as the latter can be done kindly. We may sometimes fail because illness is less bleak for this man in this situation, than health, and is the only way of life conceivable for him. Some hysterical invalidism is incurable when deeply ingrained.

Removal of symptoms by suggestion

Symptoms often disappear spontaneously as progress is made under the headings above. Sometimes however they remain, the patient being convinced that he is ill because he still feels ill, and this may not be surprising after investigations, failed treatments and medical disagreements, over a long period. It is in this situation, when relief has been afforded so far as possible but the symptoms persist, that methods of removal based on suggestion are useful. The aim is to return the patient to health naturally, without humiliation and without argument. The classical technique is hypnosis, but hypnosis is not necessary, and it can even tempt the hasty doctor to use suggestion too early, by-passing the work needed on relief of stress and psychotherapy. The hypnotist might then deal with the symptoms successfully (and this is crucially useful if it restores communication with a hysterically deaf, mute or amnesic patient) only to find others replace them later because the patient still cannot face his stress (see Case No 1, page 38). When the situation is ready for the removal of symptoms, any impressive treatment, tactfully applied, may be as effective as hypnosis: success has been achieved by a definitive physical examination, liniment, physiotherapy and manipulation, nasty-tasting medicine, nice-tasting medicine, one X-ray photograph or E.C.G., or even a well-judged wink from a family doctor.

References and Further Reading

Freud and Breuer's *Studies in hysteria* of 1895, translated and reprinted in Pelican Freud Library Volume 3, 1974, contains extremely vivid and readable case-histories and much profound speculation on the condition. Different modern viewpoints can be found in E. Slater, 'Diagnosis of hysteria', in *British Medical Journal* 1965, *1*, 1395–9 (many organically ill patients; is sceptical about the concept of hysteria) and C. Rycroft 1970, in *Anxiety and neurosis*, Harmondsworth: Penguin.

Chapter 10

Obsessive-Compulsive Reaction

DEFINITION

These are mental experiences, ideas, images, impulses or patterns of behaviour in which a subjective sense of compulsion is opposed by a conscious and deliberate resistance. They are usually repetitive, often unpleasant, always unwelcome, and accompanied by emotional tension.

By convention, the terms obsession and compulsion, when used alone, are usually reserved respectively for the mental preoccupation on the one hand and the urge to perform, as well as the actual performance of, the ritual act or pattern of behaviour, on the other. In practice, they are usually both encountered in the same syndrome.

AETIOLOGY

The capacity to develop an obsessional preoccupation, for example with a tune in the head, or a senseless idea which recurs repeatedly, is perfectly normal. The tendency is increased by fatigue or anxiety, and it is in this sense that the condition is referred to as a reaction to the stress of anxiety. A specific vulnerability to the development of this pattern of mental activity, to the extent that it becomes recognizable as an illness, has a strong constitutional basis; and this is to some extent hereditary. As in so many other forms of mental illness, the hereditary factor can also produce an environmental contribution. The parent from whom the patient acquires the genetic background will also have influenced the patient's early life by example and upbringing.

Obsessive-compulsive patterns of thought and behaviour are also apt to be released by damage to the brain; and so are seen in some cases following head injury, and also following encephalitis. For example, post-encephalitic parkinsonism is frequently accompanied by obsessive-compulsive symptoms as well as by oculogyric crises.

CLINICAL PICTURE

The symptoms may be general and diffuse, or, more frequently, related to one of a limited number of specific preoccupations. When general and diffuse they represent a pathological meticulousness which affects every aspect of the individual's life. They are particularly associated with difficulty in finally completing any activity. For example, the patient cannot turn off a tap without returning several times to turn it on again, and then off, to make sure that it is properly turned off. Letters cannot be posted without the envelope having been opened and resealed a number of times, sometimes a specific number such as 3, 7, 9 (three times three), 11, and so on. The day-to-day business of getting up, getting dressed, going to work, completing routine tasks, and returning home, may become quite impossible, because the time taken to check and re-check each stage of each procedure, often complicated by having to do things in a certain prescribed and extremely complicated way, may delay completion even of the morning dressing and toilet until it is time to start going to bed. For example:

Case No. 20
One patient of this kind took 2½ hours to shave, much of this time being taken up in checking the exact setting of the razor, in making sure that all the adjustable parts were screwed to a particular degree of perfect balance and tension. Similarly when punching a card either to clock in or to clock out at work, the card had to be taken back six to a dozen times to make quite sure that it had been properly punched, and that the time and date upon it corresponded accurately with the actual hour and day on which the operation had been undertaken.

Specific preoccupations which become the centre of obsessive compulsive rituals are usually:

> *Sexual* connected with a fear of impregnating women, if the patient is a man, or of becoming pregnant, if the patient is a woman, or

aggressive   connected with a fear of causing injury or doing
                 harm, including to the patient himself, or
contaminatory connected with a fear of conveying or acquiring
                 infection or contamination by handling material
                 from which dirt or germs may be picked up,
                 either to harm the patient, or more frequently
                 to be passed on by the patient to other people
                 who will then be harmed by them.

Tidiness, to control disorder, is often connected with thoughts of
avoiding harm to people (who might trip over untidy things) and
avoiding contamination by cleaning away dirt, as well as inspiring
a feeling of safety. The themes may be combined: sexual and
aggressive themes as in obsessional thoughts of rape; sexual and
contaminatory themes when the preoccupation is with the possible
transmission of venereal disease.

These preoccupations lead to extremely complicated and vexa-
tious rituals expressly designed to avoid the contingencies expressed
by the fears. For example, an obsessional man may be compelled
to wash the bath out with disinfectant three or four times, before
taking a bath, then again after taking a bath, to avert contamination or insemination of the bath or bathwater which then might
infect or impregnate the next woman to take a bath in the same
tub. Such fears are in no way mitigated by their recognition as
senseless and irrational.

It is absolutely characteristic that the patient knows full well
the futility both of the ideas, and of the measures which he feels
compelled to take to reduce the anguish which they cause him.
Not only has he insight, but he is even more keenly aware of the
absurdity of his predicament, and intolerant of its repercussions on
his life than are those in whom he may be tempted to confide.
He is in fact more angry about the senseless suffering which he
inflicts upon himself and others than they are.

The syndrome shows a very marked tendency to develop eventually into a conditioned reflex, whereby the association of the
painful idea with the ritual of thought or action necessary temporarily to dispel it, becomes finally completely unrelated to logic or
reason of any kind; so that, for example:

Case No. 21

A highly intelligent woman who had obsessive fears about pregnancy, eventually contrived to undergo a hysterectomy at the age of forty-five, partly in the hope that this would finally dispose of her fear of becoming pregnant by contact with articles which might at some earlier stage have been handled by a man. But in fact, after the operation she found that her rituals of glove-wearing, hand-washing, and total inability to deal normally with household chores, were quite unaffected by the fact that she no longer had a uterus, and therefore could not under any circumstances become pregnant. She had to perform exactly the same rituals in order to reduce the anguish which arose in exactly the same way. 'This proves to me', she said, in an agony of fury and despair, 'that I am completely mad'.

PSYCHOPATHOLOGY

Whereas hysterical symptoms represent t'.e effects of formation of a symbolic concept, with powerful emotional associations, at an essentially unconscious level of mental activity, obsessive-compulsive symptoms represent the formation of a symbolic concept with comparably powerful emotional associations, initially at a conscious level. The anxiety related to this is also fully recognized and acknowledged by the patient, although its intensity is inexplicable and distressing. The rituals represent a regression to a primitive magical level of thinking, whereby manipulating an idea, or carrying out a motor act in a certain way, gives a subjective feeling of power or control over an otherwise threatening situation. So hand-washing attempts symbolically to wash away the taint of guilt, as in the cases of Pontius Pilate and Lady Macbeth, who had deaths on their consciences. The ritual, while comforting, remains irrational, like the feeling which it is invoked to control.

A less momentous example is seen in childhood, when a child walks on the lines of the pavement, in order to secure some kind of favourable alteration in the pattern of the day's events. An example of rituals as a response to anxiety and as a way of coping with it, was given in Chapter 8 in describing the normal state of candidates before an examination: front-doors, pens and shoelaces are on that particular day checked several times by those with constitutional obsessional tendencies. The later stage of consolidation of symptoms, whereby the stimulus-response reaction becomes automatic and virtually a conditioned reflex, in no way mitigates the distress, but may make the syndrome even more powerfully established, and its complication and ramifications even more widespread. Ultimately, although insight is retained, the patient's capacity to control behaviour in the light of it may be totally lost.

It is necessary to recognize that the compulsively obsessional personality is not necessarily pathological. Exceptionally meticulous people may owe their perennial concern with precision and exactitude to an elaborate defence mechanism in their personality to avoid error, carelessness or catastrophe. Such meticulousness may be extremely necessary, particularly in professional men with a great responsibility for accuracy, and it may distinguish the most successful, as well as being a hallmark of the bank official or railway signalman. It is a question of assets and drawbacks in different fields: the controlled, organized and reliable man will be good value as a bank clerk but not a success in a job requiring quickness, creativity and the artistic temperament; and the converse is equally true.

In the psychodynamic hypothesis, obsessional-compulsive symptoms are seen as defences against unconscious threats, the anxiety tending to have roots in infancy and particularly in primitive aggression at the period when the infant is supposed to experience sensual pleasure from defaecation. These forbidden pleasures are warded off by obsessional phenomena, but typically the repressed themes and desires nevertheless return deviously and in disguise to conscious life, *in the content of the symptoms*. The man preoccupied with being exquisitely clean nevertheless selects a series of very dirty jobs, studies his stools in great detail and smears himself, albeit with soap, many times a day; the man who is so greatly distressed by thoughts of harming his beloved wife, does in fact exhaust and so hurt her by frequently reporting his distress to her.

The common theme is that obsessional-compulsive phenomena, the thoughts and the rituals, are *efforts at controlling threatening emotion*, whether the internal threats of sexual and aggressive desires or the external ones of disease, dirt, disorder and uncertainty.

TREATMENT

Psychotherapy
This is most likely to be successful in a proportion of cases seen early in the development of the disorder, and particularly in children. But in its widest sense it is necessary for the acceptance,

effective aid, and comfort of all patients, who are already more than halfway towards expecting and dreading ridicule and contempt when they venture to communicate their symptoms.

Interpretive psychotherapy, especially psychoanalysis with its technique of free association, has not been successful despite the fascinating symbolic material available in what the patient says. The ponderous emotional control is usually an insurmountable obstacle to this method of freeing the patient's thoughts.

Behaviour therapy
Rituals can be extinguished and anxiety reduced by desensitization and flooding methods, as described in the treatment of phobias. In the case of handwashing rituals, the patient is encouraged to contaminate himself to the full with the avoided dirt and to refrain from washing. Either this is handled as a desensitization technique, gradually trying more and more difficult tests but avoiding evoking anxiety by relaxation, hypnosis, drugs or the rapport with the therapist; or by flooding in which maximal anxiety is faced and the ritual is forbidden or prevented, a situation felt to be inconceivable by the patient, but which he comes through with consequent breaking of conditioned reflexes and vicious circles. The treatment may need to be continued in the patient's home environment, and may have to include discussions and involvement with members of his family. The techniques can be adapted to tackle obsessional thoughts also, when the same principles apply. It is of course always essential that the patient understands what is intended in the treatment and that his agreement be not only voluntary but whole-hearted.

Drug treatment
Anxiety may need to be reduced directly with tranquillizers such as diazepam, the use of which is described in Chapter 8, and tricyclic antidepressant drugs, described in Chapter 7, relieve underlying depressive illnesses, which account for some fluctuations in obsessional syndromes.

E.C.T.
Sometimes E.C.T. is used in similar circumstances, to treat accompanying depression.

Psychosurgery

Intractable tension and anguish, unrelieved in any other way, may rarely call for consideration of one of the modern psycho-surgical operations, which obtain good results in the relief of the tension itself and therefore afford an opportunity to renew other methods of treatment vigorously.

PROGNOSIS

Of cases seen within six months to a year of onset, about 15–20 per cent may respond to a combination of psychotherapy and medical measures, and perhaps another 20 per cent to E.C.T. Surveys of the state of series of patients up to twenty years later show about three-quarters unchanged and one quarter much improved. Patients with the typical syndrome, without significant depression, and with no hint of psychosis, tend to have had an early onset of symptoms and to have a poor prognosis with few remissions and few improvements.

References and Further Reading

The classical psychoanalytic case-study is Freud's account of 'The Rat-man'. Clear discussion is found in A. J. Lewis 1967, *Inquiries in psychiatry* (pp. 157–72 on 'Obsessional illness'), Routledge and Kegan Paul, and detailed accounts of series of patients by E. Kringlen, 'Obsessional neurotics: a long-term follow-up', in *British Journal of Psychiatry* 1965, *111*, 709–22; J. Pollitt, 'Natural history of obsessional states: a study of 150 cases', in *British Medical Journal* 1957, *1*, 194–8 (reprinted in the Wyeth compilation of classical papers); and J. Pollitt, 'Obsessional states', in *British Journal of Hospital Medicine* 1969, *2*, 1146–51 (reprinted in *Contemporary psychiatry*, T. Silverstone and B. Barraclough (eds), British journal of psychiatry special publication No. 9, 1975).

Chapter 11

Immaturities of Personality

PSYCHOPATHIC PERSONALITY

DEFINITION

Psychopathic personality represents a failure of maturation of personality whose impact is evident not so much in the mind or feelings of the patient as in his conduct, and particularly in his failure to make an effective adjustment to the rest of society. This is the fundamental abnormality of the psychopath, and although characteristically independent of any degree of intellectual impairment, it corresponds in terms of personality development to a failure to emerge from the explosive period of early infantile development. The psychopath has not matured emotionally beyond the age of four or five.

The failure of social development may be accompanied by signs in related fields. The E.E.G. record tends to be dominated by waveforms of frequency and distribution normally seen in children below the age of five. The psychological attitudes, no less than the personal history and day-to-day behaviour of the psychopath, remain understandable on a basis of explosive childishness rather than by postulating any other kind of abnormality of adult functioning.

In the Mental Health Act of 1959 the definition, a relatively wide and non-specific one, is: 'psychopathic disorder means a persistent disorder or disability of mind (whether or not including subnormality of intelligence) which results in abnormally aggressive or seriously irresponsible conduct on the part of the patient, and requires or is suspectable to medical treatment'. A rider adds that this definition is not satisfied if the only disorder is promiscuity or other 'immoral' conduct. There is no such legal category in Scotland.

The condition is not 'mental illness'. It is marked variation of personality, and although it may be very extreme, handicapping to the patient, and especially disastrous to those around him and to society at large, minor degrees of irresponsibility of personality shade off into the normal without sharp boundaries.

AETIOLOGY

Hereditary, constitutional and environmental factors, both in early childhood and later, have been invoked. The hereditary component is difficult to assess, resting largely on the similarly of types of personality in identical twins, and where present is likely to be related to multifactorial genes. Together with the constitutional element it may account for the occasional emergence of psychopathic personality in one member of the family when parental relationships and the siblings are apparently normal. E.E.G. and other psychophysiological findings confirm the presence of physical differences in many cases.

The part played by brain damage is probably very small, although occasional convincing cases are found. In epilepsy, Pond's studies show that delinquency is more related to poor social background than to the epilepsy. Prematurity seems not to handicap intelligence or personality development.

There is a good deal of evidence on the part played by family and social attitudes in childhood. Psychopaths, with monotonous, appalling frequency come from broken homes. Not only are the parents often uninterested and loveless, but naked hostility has in many families been the lot of the youngster who grows up into a psychopathic personality. These general findings disguise a very variable resistance in different individuals to different parental attitudes. Wider social factors are involved too, in that in some sections of society the prevailing sub-culture can involve normal training in antisocial attitudes, criminal interests and selfish brutality to people in one's path, and in other places it may be normal for most families to offer very little systematic training in social conformity to their children.

Craft summarises the evidence on causation as pointing 'to a genetic endowment for type of personality trait, to the quality of early childhood care for its strength and direction, to brain damage for exacerbation of existing traits (and the addition of frontal lobe irresponsibility or temporal lobe induced emotional outbursts depending on the site of damage), to adverse environmental pressures deepening personality traits to a psychopathic degree, and chance local factors allowing the crisis to develop that brings the individual to attention'.

CLINICAL FEATURES

The positive features include first a *lack of positive feeling or love towards others*, and secondly a liability to *act on impulse and without forethought*. Further consequences are that a loveless impulsive person may be *aggressive* to others in suitable circumstances, and may seem to be *lacking in shame or remorse* for his harmful actions. Typically he has shown inability to profit by or use experience, which includes a lack of response to punishment, and this is often reflected in a history of criminal convictions in childhood, youth and early manhood. This, with a lack of drive or motivation leads to a general *inadequacy* of conduct, so that he does not use his apparent abilities, is vulnerable to disaster when under stress and repeatedly *yields easily to the temptation of immediate irresponsible pleasure* from drugs, drink, sex, gambling, stealing or losing his temper. Negative features in the diagnosis are the absence of psychosis, the absence of severe intellectual deficit, and the lack of criminal motivation or of planning of actions in the light of the risks at issue.

The psychopath can be regarded as falling between the insane and the criminal. He is recognizable as 'the black sheep of the family'. At one time he was sent abroad to become a remittance man, paid to keep away from his respectable relatives; nowadays he may attempt to solve his problems by crime, sponging on family or living on Social Security, and frequently ends up in prison. Psychopaths are essentially people who seem completely unable to live on ordered terms with society: their inadequacy or irresponsibility or badness is part of a true disability for which we have no wholly satisfactory treatment.

They tend to be explosive personalities with a very low tolerance for stress. They may display tantrums, sulks or running away as patterns surviving from childhood, when they cannot cope with the situation.

Case No. 22

An example was a young man who landed himself in a military prison on the eve of being commissioned because he masqueraded as an officer two days before he actually would have become one, simply to impress a casual acquaintance. His father was an eminent retired military man, and the patient was his only son. He had never been able to make very much contact with his father, but respected him from a distance. He idolized his mother, but remarked 'I am afraid I am a great disappointment to her. . . .'

The circumstances of his presenting difficulty were that he had met a girl in a bar in the town where his barracks were situated, who had challenged his quite honest contention that he had been selected for commission. He had gratuitously boasted that he would meet her in the same bar the following evening and prove the truth of his contention. That night he had broken into the Quartermaster's Store, stolen the shoulder badges appropriate to second lieutenant, and appeared wearing them the following evening at the bar where his girl friend was due to meet him. She failed to turn up, and he was arrested by the Military Police.

Discussing the episode afterwards, which had cost him the commission, and had been followed by his again masquerading as an officer off duty and passing dud cheques, he said 'I can't think why they make all this fuss about it. They knew I was due to be an officer; and the banks should know that my father would see the cheques were honoured if they had only paid them for me. . . .'

Psychopaths want what they want immediately; whatever the consequences. They seem unable to postpone gratification for the sake of future stability or success. They may be intelligent or dull; but are especially inadequate in sustaining social relationships; and they tend to work out their problems on their environment, rejecting medical or psychological help except as an emergency measure in extreme crises. Even then they will exploit such help rather than cooperate with it if they can. They appear to have strong inner demands, and are emotionally intractable. They act on impulse, attempt to live out their fantasies, and very rarely display foresight or wisdom. They attempt instead to distort and misinterpret reality to make it fit their own self-centred concepts.

Their resulting lives are always unsuccessful. The inadequate psychopaths, especially after leaving parental shelter, if only in middle age, become the typical long-term clients of the social workers with 'multiple social problems'; the aggressive psychopaths receive ever longer prison sentences; all will have an unstable work record, with very many jobs held very briefly.

Case No. 23

A man of twenty-four with eight previous convictions, whose present offence, for which he was serving a sentence of five years' imprisonment, was shooting at a policeman in the course of a house-breaking attempt. This man's personal history included three admissions to mental hospitals for suicidal attempts. Of his relationship with his father he remarked, 'I don't speak to my father; he killed my mother . . .' By this he meant that his mother died as the result of a criminal abortion which his father insisted she should procure. His school and job record were characterized by frequent changes; and his response both to punishment and to appeals was to become acutely tense and uneasy, and to try in his own words 'to break out, to get away, to hide out'.

His one solace was painting. In the course of examination he repeated over and over again, 'I'd be all right if I had my paints. . . . Why won't they let me use my paints . . ? If I can't do that I'll have to do something else'. An example of 'something else' which he felt compelled frequently to 'do' was to leap into the water tank while being allowed to take his exercise within the prison grounds. This simply added to his own discomfort, and everybody else's trouble, and led on more than one occasion to a violent struggle when his rescue and the removal of his wet clothes was attempted.

His destructive, impulsive, and wholly unprofitable outbursts were phenomena which, when comparatively calm, he could discuss with considerable insight. He knew he upset not only himself but everybody else and he knew that because of his behaviour it was sometimes difficult for the other prisoners to feel safe with him, or for the prison officers to allow to the whole group a degree of latitude to which they might otherwise have attained.

The repercussions of this man's behaviour and attitude were in fact disastrous for himself and for everybody else. He was a classical example of the impulsive, aggressive, explosive psychopath whose clinical rating, E.E.G. findings, and morphological state were all characteristic.

DIAGNOSIS

This is made on the above criteria manifest in the life history and the evidence of physiological and psychological immaturity already indicated. The diagnosis is reserved for adults, since ostensibly psychopathic behaviour in childhood and adolescence may subside without lifelong disturbance following.

TREATMENT

Patients with psychopathic personality rarely complain of their personality disorder as such: they are likely to seek help either for the immediate predicament in which they have become involved (for example, an ultimatum from a beaten-up wife about separation, or the danger of a long prison sentence for repeated dangerous fighting), or for the reaction which it has evoked, such as anxiety or depression.

Basically the object of treatment must be to reinforce whatever latent tendency may exist towards maturation of personality, and to provide the social training lacking earlier in life. This can sometimes be achieved by group psychotherapy; very occasionally by skilled intensive individual psychotherapy. Such individual work is liable to involve the doctor in disappointment and frustration, because often the patient will attempt to exploit the medical relationship in exactly the same way as he has attempted to exploit all other relationships throughout his life.

There are projects to improve the treatment by using special forms of group psychotherapy in a residential therapeutic community, a regime pioneered by Maxwell Jones at the Henderson Hospital. The patients are forced to form a community, sharing work and play and indeed the whole day together, learning from and tolerating each other, in an atmosphere which encourages personal responsibility for their actions in the case of all members present, however unstable. Evasions and excuses for irresponsibility are not allowed by the backslider's peers. Acceptance of responsibility is encouraged by a system of numerous posts and committees, so that authority ceases to be seen as an alien matter. Patients stay for periods of months, or over a year, and it is claimed that half of them are improved and keep out of trouble for long periods. Self-help communities with volunteers, social workers or former patients as the staff, have experimented with variations of this method, often with particularly drastic forms of confronting the patient with his evasions and irresponsibilities for long hectic sessions in front of the whole community. Successes are claimed with some very disturbed people, but comparisons are needed with more traditional custodial and authoritarian institutions, for close study of the results of Borstal and its after-care supervision suggests that this can also claim creditable results.

Some psychopaths are cared for in secure conditions in the

Special Hospitals such as Broadmoor and Rampton under orders of the Mental Health Act or after conviction for offences. The Butler report on Mentally Abnormal Offenders, after noting that most psychiatrists did not claim to have successful methods of treating psychopaths, recommended the setting-up of training units within the penal system for dangerous anti-social patients, with a flexible regime of appropriate work and social activity.

PROGNOSIS

In general, intervention in a crisis is more successful than efforts to change the personality. Severe psychopathy is seen less often in middle age and later, although the reason for this is not certain: it may be that the personality matures by its own inner processes, or there may be some learning taking place, however slight, from the experiences of life, but it could be, more tragically, that they are, many of them, sequestered in prison for long sentences. The frustrations are not a reason for refusing to try to help psychopaths, since in their variety, pathos, and sporadically savage or helpless lovelessness, these people constitute a formidable challenge, not simply to medicine, but to mankind.

HYSTERICAL PERSONALITY

DEFINITION

Hysterical personality is the outcome of a failure of maturation less profound than that of psychopathic personality, but nevertheless sufficiently marked and definite to constitute a basic psychological syndrome. Whereas the psychopath's emotional development has remained infantile, the patient with hysterical personality has reached the stage of childhood but has failed to emerge from adolescence. Once again, this failure of emancipation from a childhood relationship with parents and the rest of the world, is quite unrelated to intelligence.

AETIOLOGY

As with psychopathic personality, constitutional and environmental factors are both important. In the environmental contribution, the key factor appears to be an incomplete and very often deeply divided emotional relationship to one or both parents, characteristically the parent of the opposite sex. It is as though the patient had failed to complete the part of the growing-up process whereby the child's dependence upon the parent is replaced by adult respect and regard. The patients show childlike, submissive and apparently defeated attitudes in positions imposing stress and requiring responsibility. They attempt at times to gain control of people by emotional manipulation rather than entering into adult negotiations and relationships. In America the term 'passive/aggressive' personality is often used.

CLINICAL FEATURES

The person with a hysterical personality tends to be characterized on the psychological side by an outgoing extroverted attitude, a relatively good capacity to make superficial contact with other people, a histrionic type of behaviour with a strong tendency to dramatization, and a measurably high degree of suggestibility. On the physical side there may be evidence of immaturity also. People of this kind, therefore, tend to be both over-demanding and yet shallow in their relationships to others; to display something of the irresponsibility of children towards adult decisions, and a good deal of the child's helplessness in dealing with the complications with which such irresponsibility inevitably confronts them. This is apt to be the more striking, and socially unacceptable, because of the articulateness and obvious intelligence often possessed by this type of individual. In the light of this it is understandable that such patients frequently develop neurotic reactions to the inevitably painful and infinitely complicated processes of adult emotional adjustment, for which they are not fully equipped. In sex and marriage, a characteristic finding is of a female hysterical personality, flirtatious yet frigid, emotionally tempestuous, married to a quiet, stable and undemonstrative husband. When things are going well she recognizes him as a tower of strength for her, and as 'very good, he doesn't trouble me for sex very much'. When the atmosphere in the relationship is poorer, he is reproached for timidity and diffidence, and she longs for a tougher, rougher style from him.

DIAGNOSIS

This is essentially a matter of clinical assessment, and is not difficult once the existence of this type of personality disorder is recognized. The decisive feature is the apparently incorrigible, manipulative childishness, displayed throughout the patient's entire attitude to life. Just as an insecure child plays off one parent against the other in his unconscious and desperate attempt to gain some kind of relative security, so the adult with hysterical personality contrives the same kind of manipulation between doctors, family, and friends; helplessly, almost always to his own ultimate detriment, and yet with an uncannily perceptive intuitive skill which creates its own tensions, and exploits the vulnerability of all who come into contact with the patient.

TREATMENT

This is usually required for symptoms of overt hysterical illness, anxiety or depression, arising out of the general circumstances created by such patients in their ineffectual attempts to deal with the problems of adult life. The initial impression is that here, above all, is a most suitable subject for individual psychotherapy. The combination of sufficient intelligence, rapport, apparent insight and a sincerely appealing and convincing desire for help, is apt to prove irresistible. Unfortunately, experience is a bitter guide, since the innate and constitutional element of immaturity tends ruthlessly to limit both the degree of cooperation and, therefore, the amount of progress of which such patients are capable. Supportive psychotherapy is often in the long run the best that can be offered, together with appropriate symptomatic treatment for the particular syndrome which they present on the occasion of consultation.

References and Further Reading

The best monograph is Michael Craft 1966, *Psychopathic disorders*, Pergamon, who is especially clear on definition and aetiology. Further detailed surveys of special aspects of psychopathy are P. D. Scott, 'The treatment of psychopaths', in *British Medical Journal* 1960, 1641–6; J. S. Whiteley of the Henderson Hospital, 'The psychopath and his treatment', in *British Journal of Hospital Medicine* 1970, *3*, 263–70 (reprinted in *Contemporary psychiatry*,

T. Silverstone and B. Barraclough (eds), British journal of psychiatry special publication No. 9, 1975); and T. C. N. Gibbens et al., 'A follow-up study of criminal psychopaths', in *Journal of Mental Science* 1959, *105*, 108–15. There is excellent discussion in *Report of the committee on mentally abnormal offenders* (Chairman, Lord Butler) Cmnd. 6244, H.M.S.O. 1975. A classic study of a hysterical personality in a ward is T. Main, 'The ailment', in *British Journal of Medical Psychology* 1957, *30*, 129–45.

Chapter 12

Sexual Problems

Normal Development

General aspects of psychosexual development were mentioned in Chapter 3. Some more detailed points will be made here.

Male and female sex hormones are present in individuals of both sexes, although in greatly different amounts, because of their production from the adrenal cortex as well as from the gonads. The low levels of childhood begin to increase before puberty, and in boys there is a major increase in androgens at that time. This is much less marked in girls, in whom it is the oestrogen levels that rise sharply. Puberty spans about four years, and tends to begin earlier in girls. In girls the first sign is usually enlargement of the breasts, followed by menarche, with a normal age range of the latter from 10 to 16. The commonest age of menarche, thirteen years, has been falling for a long time, although it now seems to be stationary.

Childhood sexual activity in the form of erections, genital manipulation, simple sex games and occasional masturbation, increases in frequency during the pre-pubertal period, so that the so-called 'latency' of psychoanalytic theory is true only of outward social life, not of sexual interests.

Androgens affect sexual drive in both sexes; the oestrogens seem not to affect libido but they are necessary for maintenance of a vascular and mucous vaginal lining. The development of normal adult behaviour including sexual intercourse doubtless is influenced by social factors however, from early experiences with the parents onwards.

The development of the feeling of being a sexually mature man or woman itself depends on having been brought up as a boy or girl. Studies of hermaphrodites and pseudohermaphrodites with ambiguous external organs have shown that the child grows up to feel psychologically and sexually a member of the sex to which he is assigned at birth, even if this conflicts with chromosomal sex or with the gonad present.

Homosexuality

Homosexuality occurs as a normal phase in sexual development in adolescence, and may persist into adult life as a partial or a settled and complete homosexual orientation. In heterosexual individuals it may re-appear under conditions of stress or deprivation – for example in prison or one-sex boarding schools.

Twin studies suggest that inherited factors contribute to the aetiology, and furnish a vulnerability to environmental factors during development, especially during childhood. The chromosomes and endocrine function of homosexuals are normal, although there is just a possibility that androgen failure during a crucial period of intrauterine life could be invoked as a cause in males, by preventing the formation of masculine patterns of behaviour thereafter.

The environmental factors in males are probably concerned with the relationship with the parents. Many studies suggest that the male homosexual typically had difficulty in establishing a good relationship with the father, who was often absent from the home either physically, or at least as a dominant figure. The weak fathers are dominated by their wives, who as mothers are close and overwhelmingly emotional and intimate with their sons. It could be that in such a family the son cannot mature emotionally to the stage of heterosexual desire for the female, although the further stages in developing a sexual orientation towards men are not at all clear. The theory is uncertain at the present time, and would in any case be incomplete without reference to sociological matters including the influence of attitudes of ostracism or acceptance of homosexuality in society.

Seduction into homosexuality by youthful experiences is probably rare, in both sexes, traces of impending homosexual orientation often being present in the victim before the incident.

In the female homosexual, the lesbian, the situation with regard to knowledge of the aetiology is similar: a mixture of genetic and environmental factors is involved, with a number of theories pointing to difficulties the girl has in establishing a relationship with her father, and the prospect of more knowledge of intrauterine hormonal influences in future research.

It has been estimated that about 4 per cent of adult men, and a much lower proportion of women, have been exclusively homosexual all their lives, while about 25 per cent of men and about 15 per cent of women enter upon frankly homosexual relationships at one time or another.

In the past male homosexuals often came for medical help when they were in trouble with the laws against their sexual behaviour, saying that they wanted help to change. This is now uncommon, but consultations may still be precipitated by duress in the form of pressure from parents or spouses on patients of either sex. The patient may come reluctantly as if to show them that he has truly tried to get treatment, and it will be the doctor's task to detect and understand this situation, trying to assess whether the patient really wants treatment, of his own accord, to change his orientation. It is very unusual for this to be the case, and the doctor's support may greatly help in enabling the patient to continue to live with what he feels to be the only possible way of life for himself.

Other consultations may be at times of distress when a homosexual relationship has broken up, leaving the patient in despair about his future, but understanding and support at the time of misery and guilt may help to tide the patient over to better times, when it turns out that there is no request for a major plan of treatment. Discussions on better adjustment to the insecurities and adversities of homosexual life are often what are needed.

Homosexuals are liable to the same gamut of psychotic, neurotic and personality problems as are heterosexual people, and these conditions will need to be treated in the usual ways described in other chapters of this book.

There remains a small number of patients who continue to ask for treatment to change their orientation. Specialized methods have been applied for this aim, including dynamic individual psychotherapy or psychoanalysis, and behaviour therapy techniques, formerly using crude aversion therapy, now more frequently desensitization to the anxieties perceived in the heterosexual relationship, but the results even in the hands of specialists have been poor.

Fetishism

This is the substitution of a symbolic object for the normal goal of union with a member of the opposite sex, as fulfilment of the sexual instinct. The object may be a particular part or aspect of the normal goal, such as the hair or the feet or the buttocks; or it may be more remote, for example an article of clothing. This in turn may have to be worn by the intended partner for orgasm to be possible; or in some cases orgasm may be prompted by the sight or touch of the object alone.

Fetishism is almost exclusively a male perversion, probably because projections and symbolic associations to sexual excitement normally contribute much more to male than to female instinctual patterns. Clearly there are elements of partial fetishism in all men, the extreme cases described above and in case No. 24 below, shading off through degrees of over-concern and over-excitement at the trappings of the sexual situation, to the normal. Usually the fetishistic interest can be traced back to early childhood, where its origins are obscure, perhaps rooted in important emotional experiences in a pleasurable or sexual situation, and persisting subsequently as a conditioned response with symbolic undercurrents: the fetish object is safer and less complicated than the female, providing a reassuring sexual situation and so ensuring erection.

Case No. 24

An unhappy young married woman of thirty-two came to the Outpatient Clinic with her husband, requesting a private interview. In the course of it she explained that the real object of the interview was to obtain advice about, and if possible for, her husband. He had developed an increasingly overwhelming desire to masturbate in front of a mirror, wearing a woman's plastic raincoat, but otherwise naked. He was still capable of occasional intercourse with his wife, but only if she also, otherwise naked, would wear the raincoat at the time. He had bought a number of these raincoats, ostensibly for his wife, but had become in all other ways extremely mean about clothes for her. Without a plastic raincoat, he was impotent, and incapable even of masturbation. Wearing one, or having persuaded his wife to wear one, he frequently had premature ejaculation, even when intercourse was attempted. Remonstration by his wife had been countered by her husband's threatening to leave her, and 'Hang around cinema queues on rainy nights – I'd soon pick up a girl in the right sort of coat. . . .' As it was, he found such queues almost irresistible. His wife feared that he might expose himself to suitably clad women, a fear which had led to her continued but miserable acquiescence in the domestic indulgence of her husband's fetishism.

She had predicted, quite correctly, that her husband himself would make no complaint at all; either about himself, or the sexual aspects of their married life: moreover she coupled her appeal for help for him with an earnest entreaty that while everything and anything possible should be done to cure, correct, change, or alter his way of life, nothing whatever should be said which might lead him to suppose that she herself had mentioned it.

Seen in his own turn, the husband remained blandly evasive, assuring the physician that he had come along with his wife because she was nervous about coming on her own. He implied that as far as he was concerned, the basis of consultation was her own anxiety, tension, and sleeplessness.

Successful treatment by individual psychotherapy or behaviour therapy is possible in about half the cases.

Transvestism

This means literally the wearing of clothes characteristic of the opposite sex, and in some cases may represent a special form of fetishism, in which subject and object are combined. It comes to attention mainly in men, because cross-dressing by females is more readily accepted by those around the patient and by current fashions. Usually the tendency goes back to early memories in childhood, and the patients are sometimes, but certainly not always, homosexual. The patients rarely ask to be cured; usually they come under pressure of an ultimatum from a spouse, employer or the law, or they seek non-judgmental counselling.

Trans-sexualism is the condition when a transvestite identifies himself completely with the opposite sex. Such a patient may even develop delusional convictions along these lines, maintaining that he has for instance, a truly feminine personality aberrantly imprisoned in a male body. They are nearly always physically completely normal, as are uncomplicated transvestites, but they press strongly, especially in the light of modern publicity, for hormonal treatment and for operations designed to change the anatomy of the sexual organs.

Case No. 25

A young married woman of twenty-eight who had come from an exceedingly unhappy home, and married to escape from it at the age of seventeen, came requesting amputation of her breasts. She said that after the birth of her second child, at the age of nineteen, she had been aware that she had nothing but loathing for her husband, because 'I really don't feel like a woman at all; and I didn't want to be married to a man. . . .' Her husband had been neither sympathetic nor understanding, and she had left him. She had subsequently supported herself and the two young children by going to work as a labourer, wearing man's clothes.

The basis of her present consultation was the determination to continue as a man, to 'marry' a girl friend whom she had subsequently acquired, and who knew all about her past background: but for the sake of feeling more comfortable in men's clothes, and substantiating her claim to change her whole status from that of female to male, she wanted her breasts removed and her feminine structure finally concealed. She wore her hair cut short like a man's, and spoke in a reasonable imitation of a man's voice.

Case No. 26
A man of forty-eight, balding, with normal distribution of masculine hair, including a stubble growth of beard, and absolutely normal male genitalia, requested an operation to turn him into a woman, which he knew he ought to be. His version of this operation was to have his penis and testicles amputated, and plastic operations designed to give him female breasts.

In further elaboration of his hopes and desires, he made it clear that he was proposing to seek marriage to a man when the transformation for which he longed had been completed: and said that he hoped it would perhaps not be too late for him to have a child under these circumstances.

Like many others, both these patients were seeking what was in fact a magical transformation of reality in the form of a 'change of sex' operation. It is very doubtful if the psychiatrist could ever 'recommend' such a procedure, although a very few patients have been helped in their adjustment by securing operations after years of unbroken insistence on passing as the opposite sex.

Many of these patients are highly disturbed individuals, requiring treatment for other psychiatric illness such as schizophrenia, or in great difficulties through their psychopathic personalities. Psychotherapy and aversion therapy have scarcely helped trans-sexualism itself.

Sadism and Masochism

These are pathological exaggerations respectively of the normal aggressive and submissive components of sexuality. Whenever they violate self-respect or consideration for others they constitute an indication for psychotherapy. Contrary to some expectations, sexual relationships based upon complementary characteristics of this kind are not usually satisfactory: rather indeed do they tend to be disastrous, because their mutual repercussions can prove exacerbatory, to the point of break-up or rarely to a suicidal or murderous degree.

Exhibitionism

This is a general term, which also has a specifically sexual connotation. In its general sense it can mean attention-seeking behaviour, including flamboyant self-display of any kind.

In its sexual connotation it is usually restricted to the unsolicited display of the male genitalia, which can give rise to the criminal charge of indecent exposure.

This is a common form of sexual behaviour, often compulsively repeated, with the result that the criminal record lengthens and otherwise respectable lives can be ruined. There is an association not particularly with low intelligence but with a general sexual inadequacy, many of the men being mild, passive, unsuccessful lovers, dominated by women, and either unmarried or unsuccessful in the sexual side of their marriage. Exposure shocks and frightens the female who sees it, and this seems to afford some sexual relief, sometimes with masturbation at the time, and sometimes with guilt and shame afterwards.

Court appearance deters many first offenders from repeating the offence, but those who are caught again are often sent for medical advice. Probation is often the best form of legal outcome, and although psychiatric treatment by psychotherapy only helps a proportion of the patients, there are promising experiments with group therapy and behavioural methods.

Sexual inadequacy

The account will mention feelings of *sexual inferiority*, as well as *male impotence, premature ejaculation, female frigidity* and *non-*

consummation of marriage.

These terms embrace a wide range of afflictions involving human sexual incapacity; and can in varying degrees be productive of untold personal misery and humiliation.

The impotent man and the frigid woman have one essential thing in common. They are both afraid. Indeed it is usually fear which underlies their failure, and inhibits erection in the male and a relaxed pelvic floor and patulous vagina in the female; while in every instance failure increases their guilt, despair and further anxiety. This vicious circle is as true of conscious and superficial sources of guilt, apprehension, and feelings of inferiority, as it is of deeper psychodynamic complexes, which may be inaccessible to conscious introspection and to which so much attention is necessarily paid in the more advanced treatises on this subject. On the other hand, the practitioner can nearly always offer help of great value to the large number of cases in which the source of guilt, apprehension or feelings of inferiority is reasonably superficial.

INVESTIGATION AND TREATMENT

The first essential is to make the patient feel that the doctor has time and is interested to listen to the problem, and to pay attention to the patient's feelings and way of describing them without interruption. The examiner should avoid premature questioning or jumping to conclusions, and above all guard against creating the impression that he is inclined to dismiss the complaint as trivial on the one hand, or on the other that he approaches it with an attitude of defeat and despair. A really detailed case history is essential in this condition.

The first part of the history must of necessity concern itself with the patient's account of the difficulty. When this has been thoroughly elaborated by the patient, inquiries should be directed towards previous sexual development, interests and experience, and an opportunity given for the confessing of fears, failures or indiscretions in the past. Many of these fears are bound up with guilt, either about masturbation, about extra-marital adventures, or about terrifying beliefs inculcated by misguided adults during childhood, or by equally disturbed companions during school days and adolescence. There is no need to comment on the material produced at the time, at least until the history is completed, unless the patient's manifest anxiety and distress demand a certain amount of interim reassurance to enable him to continue with the interview. The final history should include a review of the patient's general background including family history and previous illnesses, and an assessment of his or her basic personality, as well as the immediate situation in which the complaint of impotence or frigidity or dyspareunia has arisen. Much of this will be familiar to the general practitioner who already knows his patient. There remains this golden rule: generally speaking, *it is not so much what the doctor tells the patient, but what the patient tells the doctor*, which brings the initial relief and confidence. Naturally, when the patient has had his or her say there will often be simple explanation, reassurance, and advice which in good time the doctor will be able to impart.

A physical examination is needed, but usually no further investigations beyond testing the urine for glucose, unless physical illness is suspected. A review of possible physical factors bearing upon the sexual disorder will include consideration of diabetes mellitus as the commonest metabolic cause of male impotence, and other endocrine diseases, as well as any other general debilitating illness. General fatigue can impair sexual function, as can a heavy intake of alcohol or drugs of addiction, and drugs used for the treatment of hypertension are a common cause of impotence and ejaculatory failure. Depressive illness may be mentioned here too, although as with the other physical factors such as fatigue and increasing age, the obvious physical explanation should not be accepted too readily without careful consideration of whether it screens underlying personal and psychological reasons for sexual difficulty. *Why* is the patient overworking and becoming fatigued, *why* is he drinking heavily, *why* is he depressed?

In the next phase of treatment, when the underlying causes of guilt, anxiety and apprehension have been ventilated, the patient will be ready to trust the doctor in whom he or she has already confided, to the extent that the doctor's advice and plan of treatment, based on a real appreciation of the nature of the problem, will be respected and will itself bring further confidence.

The patient should be told that erection, ejaculation, acceptance of penetration and female orgasm, are all intricate but perfectly natural nervous processes which normally require a period of adjustment and confidence for their perfect exercise. Relative failure or difficulty at one point is less important than the patient's realization that, given confidence, practice, and an acceptance of the situation on both sides, things will tend to come right.

In a *joint interview* with both partners mutual misunderstandings can be detected and cleared up. Ignorance of the nature of the sexual response of members of the opposite sex is common, and much help can be passed on by discussing the nature of the differences between the sexes, how the female comes slowly to the plateau of excitement and orgasm, and responds particularly to affection and the total loving relationship, how the male peak is sharper, and how his rise to the peak depends more closely on the amount of physical stimulation.

Husbands can be unnecessarily concerned if their wives do not achieve orgasm, and the wives themselves may feel inadequate simply because they believe that orgasm is necessary as a normal response. It can be explained that a proportion of women never reach orgasm in their lives, and that, so long as they enjoy sex anyway, and so long as they are happy with their partners, they are doing fine and have nothing to feel inadequate about.

Discussion of normal sexual response includes gentle discussion of foreplay and how the partners respond to each other's hopes and pleasures, and how they may fear demands, shrink from surrender and loss of control, anticipate actual pain, dread pregnancy, or on the contrary feel tense about infertility. The emphasis is shifted by the doctor from the failure to enjoy and achieve sexual success to the aim of giving pleasure to the other partner, this ensuring in one move both a caring attitude to the other and a distraction from self-absorption in his or her own problem.

The couple are told to experiment with loving foreplay before their next attendance, but only doing what does not make them feel anxious, and strictly not going on to intercourse, even when they want to. Progress is then discussed again in another joint interview, and further more advanced suggestions made for the couple to practise when they are together again. The woman is taught how gently squeezing the base of the man's glans penis when it is erect reduces the erection, so that judicious repeated use of this manoeuvre can help to prolong the state of excitement. Different coital positions are explained to the couple, including the position with the woman uppermost kneeling astride and facing the supine man. In this position she is able to lower herself gradually on to the erect penis, tempering her own and her partner's anxieties for the progress of their lovemaking. Actual intercourse is still forbidden in these early stages, on the instruction of the doctor, to allow anxieties over the final test to recede, while sexual desire may be expected to build up during the discussions and experiments, sometimes so much so that the rules are surreptitiously but gleefully broken, and the couple report successful intercourse at their next consultation.

In the full version of treatment along these lines pioneered by Masters and Johnson, two therapists are used, one male and one female. The male therapist takes his history from the man, the female therapist from the woman, and in a joint interview between the four people, misunderstandings and fears are discussed, anxieties being allayed by each patient's having an advocate of the same sex to help him explain his difficulties. Many modifications of this original method are being tried and it may well be that simpler techniques with one doctor will obtain equally good results.

Premature ejaculation in the male, before or rapidly after penetration, is increasingly found distressing and brought as a problem for help. In severe degree it is clearly a failure of sexual function, whereas quick ejaculation after penetration may be a state of reflex conditioning to rapidity of reflex response, brought about by factors in the individual's past life, and by social mores according to which it was in some circles thought unimportant for the male partner to take slow patient loving care to bring the female to the excitement of orgasm.

Premature ejaculation can usually be relieved by the methods described above of full history-taking, discussions with the couple and instructions for sexual experiments at home, including the squeeze technique. Sometimes further help can be given by use of the drug thioridazine (Mellaril) in doses of about 50 mg before intercourse: it has an autonomic effect of partially delaying ejaculation, and some successes with the use of the drug may break the vicious circle of apprehension and failure.

Severe frigidity with vaginismus and even *non-consummation of marriage*, may respond to an admixture of gentle techniques of physical exploration combined with the indispensable psychotherapeutic methods. Best undertaken by a woman doctor, this involves very gentle exploration of the vagina by the gloved finger, discussing and relieving anxieties the while, and this may well be followed by the same procedure in the presence of the husband. Further progress can be obtained by graded dilators, encouraging the patient to use them herself.

Treatment of severe anxiety with tranquillizing drugs before the possibility of intercourse may help reduce disabling tension without inhibiting desire or performance. This can be achieved with diazepam 5 mg one to two hours before the event. Alcohol has always been tried by the patient before medical aid has been sought, and it rarely helps a serious sexual problem.

Treatment along the lines described in the above pages presupposes, of course, that whatever the outstanding problems between the partners, the patient who has come for help is prepared and willing to make whatever other efforts are necessary to solve them. It is, for example, unpropitious, to say the least, to attempt to treat impotence in an unfaithful husband if he proposes to continue the infidelity which is itself the source of his guilt towards his wife. Here the practitioner may count on at least some degree of appreciation of the real needs of the situation if he has preceded his advice by the careful attention and initially uncritical acceptance of the history when it was first given to him. Thereafter he should offer further interviews on a basis of dealing with the patient's day-to-day feelings about the problem, clarifying any residual doubts or misgivings, and receiving an account from the patient of his progress as time goes on.

A few patients presenting with complete primary impotence or vaginismus, with inability to consummate any sexual relationship from the time of their first efforts to try, will be found to have deep-laid emotional disturbances on the subject, and to be incapable of complete improvement with treatment on the above lines. For these people a plan of psychoanalytically-orientated psychotherapy over a long period may be needed.

Over the whole subject of sexual inadequacies, at least a quarter to a third of patients can be relieved in the course of perhaps six to a dozen interviews, within two or three months.

Morbid jealousy

Jealous preoccupations, tormenting with doubt and sometimes leading to desperate and tragic outcomes, are well-known in literature, and in the consulting room of the doctor who listens to his patients' confidences. The preoccupations are based on sexual insecurity and inadequacy, sometimes acknowledged by the patient, but capable of being intense and yet not fully conscious. The feelings can be projected on to the partner who then, in the eyes of the patient, becomes sexually traitorous and despicable in contrast to his own fidelity. Jealous accusations may escalate into torrents of non-stop nagging and bullying to extract a confession, or brooding resentment can lead to dangerous or murderous attacks. The search for proof becomes fanatical, with 'evidence' being found in the form of hairs and invisible marks on bed-linen, signals detected when curtains move in the house opposite or cars slow down as they pass. Delusions of infidelity may preoccupy the patient, detectable on internal evidence of his mental state, regardless of the actual blamelessness or otherwise of the accused spouse.

The syndrome occurs in a variety of psychiatric disorders, and accurate diagnosis is highly important. Some patients are suffering from schizophrenic psychosis, others from depression of psychotic intensity. Occasionally the picture is found early in a cerebral disease which will progress to dementia. An association with severe alcoholism is known, probably when paranoid features in the personality are compounded by sexual failure brought on by the alcohol, and the wife's disinclination for a sexual relationship with the frequently drunken husband. Commonly however, the condition arises in the context of a personality disorder in the patient, with immature and insecure traits inflamed in a particularly disturbed marital relationship.

Psychiatric disorders found need their own treatment as described elsewhere in this book. Psychotherapy rarely helps to change the condition fundamentally, although counselling of either partner may be needed, including advice to the target of the accusations not to 'confess' for the sake of peace when she is in fact innocent. Separation for the sake of safety has to be considered.

References and Further Reading

'Normal psychosexual development', by M. Rutter, *J. Child. Psychol. Psychiat.* 1971, *11*, 259–83, is essential reading.

Three comprehensive reviews are 'Homosexuality in the male', by J. H. J. Bancroft, in *Brit. J. Hosp. Med.* 1970, *3*, 168–81; 'Homosexuality in the female', by F. E. Kenyon, in *Brit. J. Hosp. Med.* 1970, *3*, 183–206; 'Indecent exposure and exhibitionism', by F. G. Rooth, in *Brit. J. Hosp. Med.* 1971, *5*, 521–33; all reprinted in *Contemporary psychiatry*, T. Silverstone and B. Barraclough (eds), British Journal of Psychiatry Special Publication No. 9, 1975. Transvestism and trans-sexualism have been studied especially by

J. B. Randell, see *British Medical Journal* 1959, (ii), 1448-52.

On impotence, a fuller account is by D. Stafford-Clark 1954, 'The etiology and treatment of impotence', in *Practitioner*, *172*, 397. Most of the recent developments are strongly influenced by Masters W. H. and Johnson V. E.. 1970, *Human sexual inadequacy* London: Churchill, which should be read, although with due allowance for different conditions in this country. See also H. S. Kaplan, 1974 *The new sex therapy*, London: Cassell, especially chapters 7-14.

'Morbid jealousy: some clinical and social aspects of a psychiatric symptom', by M. Shepherd, *Journal of Mental Science* 1961, *107*, 687-753, reviews the subject thoroughly; it is reprinted in the Wyeth compilation of papers.

There is much wisdom and good writing in *Sexual deviation* by A. Storr, Penguin, 1964.

Chapter 13

Psychosomatic Reactions and Kindred Syndromes

DEFINITION

Psychosomatic reactions may be defined as structural changes significantly related to emotional factors.

AETIOLOGY

In essence every form of illness to which human beings are subject has its psychosomatic aspects. In fact the essential link between psychiatry, general medicine, surgery and obstetrics, lies in the ultimate impossibility of treating states of mind apart from states of body, and states of body apart from states of mind. Had psychiatry made no greater contribution to the balance of the general medical curriculum than to endorse and emphasize this single fact, its contribution would still be invaluable; for it has all too often been the assumption in the past that, while bodily states have to be exhaustively observed and meticulously studied, mental states can be either taken for granted or dismissed as irrelevant, in the training of the doctor.

The anatomico-physiological basis for psychosomatic reaction is, on reflection, self-evident. The central nervous system, the autonomic nervous system, and the neuro-endocrine system, whose pivotal centre can be regarded as the pituitary gland, represent three inter-related systems of communication whereby the individual maintains equilibrium between himself and his external environment, and within his own organism.

The cerebral cortex and the central nervous system are primarily responsible for mediating subjective experience and objective behaviour. The autonomic nervous system is responsible for maintaining internal physiological equilibrium, and relating it to the demands of external experience. The link between the autonomic nervous system and the neuroendocrine system is provided by the neural stalk of the infundibulum which links the hypothalamus to the pituitary gland.

The various phenomena of emotion, which may be defined as a combination of subjective experience and objective physiological change, provide a normal and universal example of psychosomatic reaction. Anxiety, for instance, may arise in relation to external experience or internal cortical association in the central nervous system, as when one turns one's thoughts to a frightening topic. It will be mediated through autonomic activity in the adrenergic response, and if sufficiently long maintained, may produce changes in the neuro-endocrine system, for example in overactivity of the thyroid gland.

Although interaction between these systems is a constant and invariable aspect of human health and sickness, it tends all too often to be ignored in the practice of medicine. But in reality the repercussions of protracted fear or frustration upon physical health are not only apparent but clearly inevitable. Nor can the validity of purely subjective experience be disregarded; yet it is still possible to hear medical students and doctors talking about such meaningless and self-contradictory concepts as 'imaginary pain'; or discounting the emotional repercussions of serious physical illness.

Pain is essentially a subjective experience; either it exists or it does not. If a patient says he is suffering from pain, either he is telling the truth, or he is lying. In the first instance, his suffering is real, whether or not the doctor can find a structural explanation for it; in the second, his complaint is a form of malingering; but this is not the same as suffering from pain of functional or hysterical origin. Malingering, in contrast to hysterical symptoms, is very uncommon in general clinical practice.

SOME SPECIAL CLINICAL EXAMPLES

Examples of syndromes in which the contribution of the emotional component of the patient's experience is frequently of particular importance, include the following conditions (in some, such as hay fever, the structural changes are minimal, while impotence and dyspareunia do not figure in classical lists of psychosomatic conditions, but they are deliberately included in this list):

1 *In the cardiovascular system*
Hypertension
Angina pectoris
Ischaemic heart disease
2 *In the digestive system*
Chronic dyspepsia, colitis, both mucous and ulcerative, and the
   irritable bowel syndrome
Peptic ulceration
3 *In the skin*
Urticaria
Eczema
Possibly psoriasis and seborrhoeic dermatitis
4 *Allergic reactions and specific sensitivities such as*
Hay fever and allergic rhinitis
Bronchial asthma
Migraine
5 *In the musculo-skeletal system*
Rheumatoid arthritis
Backache, 'rheumatism', 'fibrositis'.
6 *In the metabolic and endocrine system*
Diabetes mellitus
Hyperthyroidism
7 *In the reproductive system*
Impotence – see Chapter 12
Dyspareunia and Vaginismus – see Chapter 12
Menstrual disorders
Menopausal symptoms
8 *Anorexia nervosa*

These complaints tend to have in common the importance of
the contribution of the autonomic nervous system in their development. The factor which they share is the large part which continued
or recurrent emotional stress appears to play in producing, maintaining, and influencing their course.

The example of diabetes mellitus is aptly illustrative. It has
long been known that certain disasters change the insulin tolerance
and therefore the entire equilibrium of the stabilized diabetic.
Chief among these are infection, and physiological shock associated
with injury, or with operation under anaesthesia; but an equally
significant factor can be emotional disaster.

Sudden bereavement, the infidelity or desertion of a husband or wife, or even the collapse of a business or the loss of a fortune, can precipitate diabetic coma in a previously stabilized diabetic, not by neglect of the self-administered insulin injections at such a time (although this is a possibility), but in precisely the same way as infection or other physiological disturbance. There are several relevant possible mechanisms: adrenal medullary hormones secreted during action of the autonomic nervous system are hyper-glycaemic in action, as are adrenal cortical hormones, secreted during all forms of stress, including strong emotion.

It seems that underlying a finding of this kind is an innate consistency of response of living creatures to all they have to endure, whether it be fear or pain, hunger or infection, emotional stress or physical disease.

CLINICAL IMPLICATIONS

These are simply that in taking a history and conducting an examination of the patient attention must be paid to the entire life situation of the person concerned, to his background and personal history, as well as to his presenting complaint.

One valuable and illuminating way of arranging the data thus obtained is by constructing a *life chart* for the patient. This consists of four vertically ruled columns, the first and second of which contain the date and the age of the patient throughout the life history, the third the circumstances of his life and development at the relevant times, and the fourth the symptoms from which he has suffered, including exacerbations, relapses and remissions of existent illnesses, and fluctuations in general health. Correlations which become evident in this way will enable every doctor to become a more observant, careful, effective and humane physician.

Case No. 27
Mr C. L. aet 34. Diagnosis *Ulcerative Colitis*

Age	Date	Personal History and Life Situation	Previous and Current Symptoms
Born June 17 1940			
4	March 1945	Parents separated. Patient went to residential school.	Nocturnal enuresis began.
8	October 1948	Home to mother: parents reunited – but stormily.	

Age	Date	Personal History and Life Situation	Previous and Current Symptoms
8	December 1948		Nocturnal enuresis remitted.
9	April 1950	Troubles at school. Pt. due to take scholarship. Friction between father and school teachers. Repercussions on patient.	Began missing school odd days – 'colic and diarrhoea'.
13	August 1953	Passed scholarship.	
	September 1953	Boarding school. Very unhappy.	
13	October ⎱ 1953 November ⎰		In school sanatorium with constant abdominal pain and tenesmus.
14	1954		Gradual fluctuating frequency of stools with diarrhoea over next three years.
17	1957	Left school. Unfit examinations for university. Became articled clerk to solicitors' firm.	
19	1959	Very worried re National Service. Conflicts re military service, etc. Father a regular ex-soldier: no sympathy with patient.	
19	November 1959		First noticed blood in motions.
19	December 1959	Rejected for National Service.	Symptoms remitted.
20–25	1960–65	Qualified solicitor. Mother proud. Father away.	Fit.
27	1966–67	Father returned home. Restless, unsettled, extravagant, recriminatory. Patient continued living at home. Apprehensive and resentful: contributing most of upkeep of home. Mother becoming anxious and hypochondriacal.	Relapse of bowel symptoms. Diagnosed ulcerative colitis. Refused admission hospital (could not be spared).
28	June 1968	Met serious girl friend (also with family problems). Unable to get married.	Exacerbation of ulcerative colitis. *Admitted hospital.* Symptoms subsided with rest and routine treatment.

Age	Date	Personal History and Life Situation	Previous and Current Symptoms
29	March 1970	Father diagnosed cancer of lung.	Patient very depressed: anxious, guilty. Ulcerative colitis quiescent.
30	September 1970	Father died.	Patient very upset. Health otherwise poor (insomnia – tiredness): but no active colitis.
30	April 1971	Married. Shared house with mother. Faced with involvement in problems of in-laws. Passed over for promotion in partnership firm.	
31	June 1971		Severe relapse. Ulcerative colitis. Haemorrhages. Readmitted hospital. Patient in despair and very worried. Psychiatric opinion sought.
31	July, August September 1971	Psychotherapy (interpretive and supportive) in hospital, based on material as set out.	Progressive remission to symptom-free state.
32	September 24, 1971	Discharged home. Outpatient follow-up and psychotherapy maintained (once weekly for 3 months, thereafter fortnightly to monthly review).	Insight gained. Remission continued.
34	September 1974	Three-year follow-up study.	Fit.

Case No. 28
Mrs. J. D. aet 30. Diagnosis *Rheumatoid Arthritis*

Born March 2, 1943	Only child. Devoted, anxious parents. Happy if somewhat overprotected childhood: the patient was naturally athletic, and inclined to

Age	Date	Personal History and Life Situation	Previous and Current Symptoms
		be stubborn; and had occasionally to battle with parents to be allowed to take part in 'rough games' and competitive sports at which in fact she tended to excel. Significant features in life chart emerge for the first time in early adult life and are set out below.	
24	June 1967	Married to 'headstrong ambitious young electrician of 26'.	Very well and happy.
25	January 1969	Husband determined to emigrate. Much opposition from patient's parents. Conflict and ambivalence in own mind.	Anxious, sleepless, tearful, lost weight.
26	March 1969	Mother (secretly) urged pregnancy on patient. 'Then you can delay going abroad at least a year. . . .'	Patient (guilty, and without telling husband) abandoned contraception. Previously agreed policy had been no children for first 3 years.
26	May 1969	Husband furious at deception – ('unwisely confessed' by patient under pressure).	*Became pregnant.* 'Hated self – mother – husband – unborn child . . .' Very depressed. No medical advice.
26	July 1969	Husband temporarily contrite. Mother suspicious.	*Spontaneous abortion.* Patient very upset. 'Don't know what I want. Nothing any good. . . .'
		G.P. consulted. Advised all concerned pull themselves together.	
26	September 1969	Opportunity for hubsand in Canada. Emigrated without patient: 'Too cold this time of year: you're not really fit yet: follow later when I'm settled and send for you. . . .'	Patient devastated and outraged. Blamed mother. Blamed husband. Began praying something might happen to make husband come back.

Age	Date	Personal History and Life Stuation	Previous and Current Symptoms
26	November 1969	G.P. concerned re patient's general state. Advised father to advise husband to return. Father cabled husband urgently: return at once. Husband flew back.	Patient apprehensive then relieved on seeing husband again.
26	December 1969	Husband affectionate, concerned – sex life successfully resumed. Happy Christmas at patient's parents' home.	Patient very well.
26	January 1970	Husband announced imminent return to Winnipeg: 'You can follow in spring. . . .'	Reactivation patient's distress. 'You can't leave me *again*. . . .'
		Husband's reaction 'There's nil wrong with you really: you just play up to get your own way.'	Patient humiliated and outraged once more.
26	February 1970	Husband flies back to Canada. Situation altogether strained.	Patient develops symptoms and signs rheumatoid arthritis, left wrist and hand. Symptoms remit.
		Patient discovers herself pregnant. Husband promises return to take her out to Canada in April.	Patient well and hopeful.
27	April 1970		Second spontaneous abortion. Rhesus incompatibility diagnosed. Severe rheumatoid arthritis in left wrist, hand, both knees, right ankle. Patient admitted hospital. Severely depressed. *Psychiatric consultation requested.*
		Psychotherapy instituted in light of life chart material: E.C.T. × 8 also given.	Remission and discharge in 2 months with subsequent maintenance outpatient psychotherapy for 6 months.

Age	Date	Personal History and Life Situation	Previous and Current Symptoms
27	November 1970	Contact maintained with patient and General Practitioner after further 6 months' psychotherapy.	Remission maintained.
27	December 1970	Patient flew to Canada to join husband.	
30	December 1973	Patient maintains recovery in Canada, as reported by letter in response to follow-up inquiry.	

SPECIFICITY OF CAUSES AND SYNDROMES

Despite much research effort, there are few results linking particular bodily syndromes with typical pre-morbid personalities or special problems of stress. On the contrary, the same personality descriptions tend to be quoted in a variety of psychosomatic illnesses, the typical victims being well endowed with tense obsessional drive, taking on additional obligations at work while being unable or unwilling to delegate or let up on their ambition and drive to succeed: the stereotype of the 'ulcer personality' or the colleague who is destined to have a coronary thrombosis.

What is specific is not the stress or the personality but the syndrome: the patient who as a young man develops ulcerative colitis under stress continues to have relapses of this disease under a variety of stresses throughout his life, and the same applies *mutatis mutandis* to peptic ulcer, bronchial asthma, etc.

Example: Bronchial Asthma
The syndrome of bronchial asthma, episodes of bronchial constriction in which ventilation is impeded, leading to severe dyspnoea, distress and even death, illustrates the principles of psychosomatic medicine very well. The tone of the bronchial smooth muscle is affected by many factors, both local in the bronchus, such as toxicity and irritation from obstructing purulent secretions, and distant, in the form of humoral factors, and the level of autonomic discharge. The autonomic tone is itself determined partly by the emotional state of the patient, acting via the hypothalamus. The mechanisms exist, therefore, for there to be psychological and

somatic causes, and complex mixtures of causes are indeed found in many patients.

The roles of bronchial *infection* and of *allergy*, for example allergy to the house dust mite and to certain other substances, flowers, foods and drinks, are well known, and the two factors often interact. Inhalation of the allergen is more likely to be followed by severe difficulty in breathing if there is already some infection, perhaps hardly noticed, in the bronchial lumen.

Psychological factors are frequently involved however, which is easily illustrated in the cases of many asthmatic children. The presence of the allergen becomes a conditioned stimulus to cause asthma, and sometimes the sight, or even the mention of the usual allergen will set off an attack, without any trace of its having been inhaled.

In many patients, attacks tend to be precipitated at times of emotion, although the pattern varies from one patient to another, the precipitant being sometimes frustration, sometimes resentment or fear, and even on occasion simple pleasurable excitement.

The illness can become involved in unhappy patterns of family relationships, so that, for example the patient may be likely to have an attack when there is a dispute with his mother, so that he feels angry over the row, guilty at having upset her and resentful at having been precipitated into asthma again. The mother at the same time feels angry at the row, fear and guilt at having caused another asthma attack, frustration over her inability to have a happy relationship with her delicate child, and of course tinges of other feelings too.

The mothers and other relatives have often been thought to be overanxious about asthmatic patients, encouraging complicated relationships of dependency, but this can be a harsh judgment, as well as taking insufficient account of the possibility that such anxiety as they show may not have caused the asthma in the first place, but rather be a response to the stress of having an asthmatic child.

There is no doubt that the infective, allergic and psychological causes interact, the bronchial muscle being a final common pathway. One author even supported the psychosomatic hypothesis by saying: 'asthma is certainly an allergic illness in all cases; some patients are allergic to pollen, others to their mother's apronstrings'.

The treatment comprises efforts in many different fields, logically derived from the aetiological factors. Psychiatric methods include teaching muscular relaxation, the use of hypnosis to deepen relaxation, sedation with drugs, and psychotherapy, sometimes mainly with the individual patient, but sometimes much more effective when conducted with the parents, or as family therapy.

SOME SPECIFIC CLINICAL SYNDROMES OF PARTICULAR PSYCHIATRIC IMPORTANCE

Anorexia nervosa

This is a condition in which there is a profound aversion to food, often leading to severe self-starvation, accompanied at least initially by subjective well-being and protestations of energy. Emaciation and even death from starvation or secondary infection are significant risks in untreated cases.

AETIOLOGY

The disorder is almost entirely confined to adolescent or young adult girls, although cases have been encountered occasionally in young men. Perhaps 20 per cent of cases are schizophrenic, severely depressed or suffering from an obsessive-compulsive disorder, but the typical syndrome concerns immaturity of personality and conflicts over growing up and becoming adult and sexually mature. Stormy relationships with the parents develop, if not before then during the illness. Social influences include the present-day preoccupation of young women with slimness, the rounded figure being largely out of fashion.

Anorexia nervosa often afflicts a girl in a family somewhat preoccupied with feeding and the appearance of the figure. Deliberate severe food restriction then leads to an emaciated amenorrhoeic state, in effect pre-pubertal and sexually dormant, and in the immature girl the habit is maintained for the unconscious relief this gives to sexual conflicts, as well as for other reasons such as family stress, attention, and because habits always acquire their own momentum and are difficult to dislodge.

CLINICAL FEATURES

The combination of emaciation, subjective well-being and a determined, sometimes even a desperate refusal or inability to accept a normal diet, in the absence of other primary pathology, is characteristic. Amenorrhoea is constant.

DIFFERENTIAL DIAGNOSIS

This is essentially from endocrine disorder such as hypopituitarism on the one hand and from severe latent infection, such as chronic miliary tuberculosis, on the other. The loss of secondary sexual characteristics such as pubic and axillary hair, and breast contour, is common in endocrine disorder and absent in anorexia nervosa.

TREATMENT

The first essential aim is the establishment of contact, sympathy and rapport, together with the restoration of the patient to a normal body weight and capacity for living, by a careful regime in hospital. This requires vigilant encouragement and supervision of eating by the nursing staff, with the patient in bed at first, and a prescription of chlorpromazine to help sedation and weight gain. An explicit hierarchy of rewards in return for gain in weight may be needed to start and maintain progress: only after agreed small gains in weight is the patient allowed visitors, and then permitted to get up and subsequently attend the occupational therapy department. This strict manipulation of incentives by the staff, to ensure life-saving weight-gain, needs of course to be accompanied at every stage by kind supportive contact with the patient. The second stage of treatment is attention to the underlying psychopathological problems, whatever they may be.

PROGNOSIS

Immediate prognosis in treated cases is good: long-term prognosis unfortunately bad. Over 60 per cent of patients who have suffered from anorexia nervosa either experience further attacks in later life, or display relatively crippling disorders of personality, usually on a hysterical basis.

Hypochondriasis

DEFINITION

Hypochondriasis may be defined as a morbid preoccupation with the maintenance of bodily health or the possibility of disease.

INCIDENCE

It is probably one of the commonest bugbears of general practice. In one form or another it is responsible for about 10 per cent of all regular attendances at doctors' surgeries or hospital out-patients' clinics. Subjectively it can be exhausting, humiliating and disabling for the patients concerned.

DIFFERENTIAL DIAGNOSIS

It is the importance of recognizing the underlying disorder of which hypochondriasis may be the most insistent syndrome, which merits its inclusion as a special item in this section. Hypochondriasis may in fact constitute the presenting feature of an anxiety state, or depressive illness, may represent a hysterical or obsessive-compulsive reaction, or may form part of the clinical syndrome of chronic insidious schizophrenia, or even of dementia.

ANXIETY STATES

Hypochondriasis in anxiety states can take two forms: the simpler of the two is the misinterpretation of the autonomic accompaniments of anxiety as an indication of progressive bodily disorder. This form of hypochondriasis is common in adolescence and young adults, and is particularly likely to be seen in medical and nursing students. The presenting complaints are therefore likely to be tachycardia, dyspnoea on exertion, lassitude, digestive disturbance, sweating, tremulousness, and disturbed sleep. Physical examination reveals only the autonomic accompaniments of anxiety, of which the symptoms are the outcome and not the cause.

The second variety of anxious hypochondriasis takes the form of specific phobias of particular diseases; for example cancer or venereal disease. A patient, careful and courteous clinical examination, followed by explanation and appropriately imaginative reassurance, will prove effective in some cases; but in the majority, while immediate relief and gratitude may be salutary, it is apt to be ill-sustained.

The treatment is the treatment of the underlying phobic anxiety state.

HYSTERICAL REACTIONS

Here the hypochondriasis is characteristically less charged with overt anxiety, and more with the latent need to establish an accepting and dependent relationship with another human being through the exhibition and experience of symptoms of illness. Once again diagnosis and treatment depend upon the recognition and acceptance of the underlying psychopathology.

DEPRESSION

Hypochondriacal ideas, sometimes reaching delusional intensity, are relatively common, particularly in the elderly in agitated states of depression. They have a characteristically self-punitive and nihilistic flavour: 'My bowels are blocked . . . my brains have dissolved . . . I am rotting away inside . . . I am unclean, I am not fit to be in the ward with other patients. . . .' They share the prognosis of the causal condition, and respond completely to the same treatment.

OBSESSIVE-COMPULSIVE DISORDERS

It is here that hypochondriasis is seen in its most essential form, since in many instances a morbid preoccupation with bodily health or the possibility of disease is the only way in which the obsessive-compulsive tendency manifests itself. These patients are more often men than women; often they are fussy bachelors. They may rarely trouble their doctor; being content to amass an enormous range of pills and lotions in their bathroom cupboard, and to minister incessantly to themselves in a way which brings them some comfort and solace. Sometimes anxiety and distress are not obvious, and it is as if scrutiny of their own health had become almost an obsessive hobby in an otherwise empty life. Others do persistently seek out their doctors, bringing long lists of symptoms, reporting in detail on their bowel movements and the colour of the marks on the toilet paper.

Supportive, or in suitable cases, interpretive psychotherapy is the treatment, where treatment is required.

SCHIZOPHRENIA

The characteristic of schizophrenic hypochondriasis is a bizarre delusional quality. It differs from the delusional hypochondriasis of depression in that the self-punitive, self-accusatory content is absent, while the grotesqueness of the experiences reported or the ideas expressed may exceed even those encountered in a depressive psychosis. The patients may believe in monsters inside their bodies, and feel indescribably peculiar changes and sensations, sometimes attributed to outside influences, sexual interference or persecution, and sometimes, in the patients' view, requiring surgical intervention.

Treatment once again, is that of the primary disorder, if the patient can be persuaded or enabled to accept it.

DEMENTIA

This must never be forgotten when hypochondriacal symptoms appear for the first time with a psychotic flavour in a patient in late life. The hypochondriasis of dementia is usually persistent, repetitive, bizarre, and associated at first with anxiety or woe, later with the emotional lability characteristic of the underlying disorder. Support and reassurance, although of limited duration in their effect, are always of immediate value, and often constitute a very real contribution to the relief of the patient's helpless suffering.

Reference and Further Reading

General books are *Modern trends in psychosomatic medicine*, 2, O. W. Hill (ed.), London: Butterworths, 1970, and 3, 1976.

There are two main authorities on anorexia nervosa: A. H. Crisp in an article of that title in *Hospital Medicine* 1967, 1, 713–18, reprinted in *Contemporary psychiatry* (T. Silverstone and B. Barraclough (eds), British Journal of Psychiatry Special Publication No. 9, 1975), and G. F. M. Russell in *Modern trends in psychological medicine 2*, J. H. Price (ed.), pp. 131–64, London: Butterworths, 1970.

Hypochondriasis is reviewed by F. E. Kenyon, *British Journal of Hospital Medicine*, 1976, 16, 419–28.

An excellent review is Z. J. Lipowski, 1977, 'Psychosomatic medicine in the seventies: an overview', *American Journal of Psychiatry 134*, 233–44.

Chapter 14

Alcoholism and Drug Abuse

ALCOHOLISM

Alcohol is used and prized in practically all societies, and its dangers are equally widely recognized. Drinking and drunkards make their appearance in our earliest literature, in Homer, and remain with us continuously to this day, when the enjoyment, the consumption and the disasters of alcohol are steadily increasing.

Some people can drink alcohol regularly in large amounts without becoming dependent on it and without harm to their lives, although they certainly put themselves at great hazard of dependence and damage by their heavy drinking. Dependence, as with other substances taken for their psychological effects, can be strictly physical, or psychological. Drinkers whose well-being is harmed by alcohol are alcoholics, a term which has been hard to define clearly. The usual definition is the W.H.O. one of 1952: 'Alcoholics are those excessive drinkers whose dependence on alcohol has attained such a degree that they show a noticeable mental disturbance or an interference with their mental and bodily health, their interpersonal relations and their smooth social and economic functioning, or who show the prodromal signs of such development'.

Traditional attitudes to those in trouble from drinking have been moral and legal ones, of opprobium and scorn for the inebriate, and rejection as undeserving poor for the chronic drunkard on his beam-ends. Originally the medical profession shared these views. The campaign to recognize alcoholism as an illness, therefore qualifying for the professional as well as humane concern of the health professions, has been going on for most of this century. The effect has been humane although not always logical, and problems sometimes arise when issues of personal responsibility are raised by the doctor, to be countered by the alcoholic who explains that he has an illness and cannot help it.

INCIDENCE

Surveys of populations and indirect estimates from other indices such as the death-rates from cirrhosis of the liver, are liable to many errors, but there is much agreement, first, that there are probably at least 200,000 to 400,000 alcoholics in the U.K., in fact 1 per cent of the population if early cases are included, secondly that the frequency is rising, and thirdly that the incidence is increasing especially in the young.

AETIOLOGY

There is every indication that this is highly complex, with an interplay of social, personal and physical factors in each case, not forgetting the part played by chance in bringing the different influences to bear on the individual.

Social factors include especially the place taken by social drinking, and the attitude to problematic drinking, in the life of the society. Alcohol is very differently regarded in Britain, Ireland and France, for example, and where heavy drinking is common, the individual who becomes alcoholic may not always be a highly disturbed person. The price, laws, and other factors bearing on the consumption of alcohol, have often been found to affect alcoholism rates. Some occupations are associated with heavy drinking, and inevitably, although less notoriously, with its dark side, alcoholism: traditional examples are the licensed trade at home, the Armed Services, and the Merchant Navy, but there are of course countless individual situations with relentlessly high exposure to drinking.

Personal influences on the development of alcoholism are manifest from early life onwards. Many alcoholics come from broken homes, and had experience of at least one alcoholic parent. This acts not always as a deterrent, and the force of parental example is often stronger, as the adolescent attempts to still his emotional turmoil with the same seductive drinks as did his father. Unstable personalities who demand instant pleasure and yield to the temptations of irresponsibility may become heavy and rash drinkers and eventually alcoholics, and may be joined by other people who, in the poet's phrase, cannot bear very much reality, or whose bitter cup of reality has been very full and beyond all bearing.

Heredity is not the main cause for the way that alcoholism is often passed on from parent to child, but it may play a small part. Physical factors are involved especially in the later stages of alcoholism, when physical dependency develops, with a withdrawal syndrome of sometimes great severity, and the development of physical complications of chronic repeated alcoholic poisoning, described below.

CLINICAL FEATURES

In the early stages of alcoholism drink gradually becomes, not one incidental pleasure and lubricant of social life, but a *preoccupation*, something invested with importance, something needed, something looked forward to. Later these features will become a *craving*, but early on, the signs are slight. Drink is taken every day, the quantity increases, the patient wonders how much there will be at a party, and whether it will be strong. He may start drinking alone, and with this may come the beginnings of another important feature, *guilt* about drinking. He wonders if he drinks more than he should, ponders on whether to cut it down; he deliberately cuts it out for a while, to prove his freedom from the habit. Later he will be evasive about how much he drinks, and protest, too much, that he could give it up any time if he chose to.

As he becomes alcoholic, he neglects his family, work and social obligations. Wife and children are kept short of money, and become used to seeing him drunk. Bottles of ever cheaper drinks are found around the house or in the now neglected garden. He is known as a drinker at work, sometimes is away from his post after the weekend, and he may become known to the police. Recurrent convictions for drunken driving in a normally responsible man can herald a serious drinking problem. His appetite fails, and for breakfast he takes the first drink of the day, to 'steady his nerves' and get rid of the 'shakes', a sign of physical dependence in the nervous system. 'Loss of control' may occur, the patient remaining sober for long periods, but never able to feel safe that he can pass an open pub, and never sure that once he starts drinking he will not go on, heavily, until he is drunk, disgraced and ill. Sometimes a severe alcoholic knows that something is wrong when his tolerance begins to fall; smaller amounts then make him drunk, a physical phenomenon which is not understood.

A whole series of late *complications* may occur:

Physical dependence, with tremor, restlessness and interrupted sleep when the alcohol level in the blood falls. This may lead, in cases of withdrawal from a formerly high intake of alcohol, or when the patient is physically ill, to:

Delirium tremens, with confusion, terrifying visual and auditory hallucinations, total insomnia, and a risk of grand mal epileptic fits and physical collapse.

A *chronic hallucinosis*, in the absence of confusion, may persist for weeks or months.

Physical deterioration, with hepatic inflammation or cirrhosis, peripheral neuropathy, cardiac failure of the beri-beri type, Wernicke's encephalopathy, and Korsakov's psychosis (loss of recent memory, with confabulation, while comprehension is relatively well preserved. The memory loss is sometimes permanent). Disorders of thiamine metabolism superimposed on insufficient intake of the vitamin are involved in the chemical pathology of these disorders, in combination with the long term toxic effects of alcohol.

Accidents, at work, at home or on the road.

Depression and suicide, often by mixtures of alcohol and hypnotic drugs. Suicide is a commoner cause of death in alcoholics than all the above physical complications.

Skid row: complete social deterioration, the patient becoming homeless, suffering from malnutrition and a number of physical illnesses, going in and out of prison for stealing and drunkenness, and being in danger of blindness or death in coma caused by methyl alcohol in cheap poisonous spirit.

TREATMENT

1 Education and prevention
2 Specialized service
3 Physical rehabilitation
4 Psychological rehabilitation
5 Social rehabilitation

People who may in the course of their work meet the alcoholic in the early stages of his decline, people such as family doctors, personnel officers in industry, occupational health staff and the clergy, need to be educated to probe for and recognize the prodromal signs of alcoholism, and to recognize the importance of not passing judgment. More humane and more important is to be tactful in getting him to a doctor with access to the specialized services.

Legal measures to outlaw alcohol are unlikely to be applied in this country, and are well known to have failed elsewhere, although legislation to license and control the trade here has in fact a good record of reducing the social problems and illness attributable to alcohol. It could be that legislation encouraging a closer relationship between the courts and the alcoholism service would help, if the courts could press for evidence of rehabilitation and of remission of the alcoholism of drunken offenders, before deciding on waiving or reducing punishment.

A *specialized service* is needed, for alcoholics do not do well in general psychiatric units, and special styles of work are needed in clinics and hostels in the community, with, by general agreement, a commitment to a multidisciplinary approach not only between the health professions but reaching out to the Church and voluntary organizations, who have a very creditable record in this field. A number of specialized services have been set up, and government policy is for the further setting up of detoxification centres in the front line of institutional care for the deteriorating alcoholic. After a few days in the centre, investigation and rehabilitative efforts would begin, and to have a chance of success would require access to a variety of kinds of hostel.

Physical rehabilitation of the alcoholic patient with physical complications requires an admission to hospital, investigations of liver

204 Psychiatry for Students

function and of the patient's mental state, and nursing care. Tremor, agitation and insomnia require the prescription of sedative drugs, diazepam being effective in doses of at least 30 mg daily and 10 or 20 mg at night. Large doses of thiamine, initially intravenously, should be given. Usually appetite returns in three or four days, and sleep becomes peaceful after a week or a little longer. This 'drying-out' regime can be supplemented in the case of delirium tremens, when there are hallucinations and the danger of grand mal fits, with larger doses of diazepam until the patient is sedated, or with additional doses of promazine in doses of 50 or 100 mg. If diazepam is being prescribed there is no need for barbiturates or phenytoin in the prevention of epilepsy, and there is no need to allow any intake of alcohol during this regime of treatment.

Psychological rehabilitation begins with first contact with the service, whether or not the patient is admitted to hospital. An educational style in the psychotherapy is the most useful, with practical attention to the weaknesses of personality and the problems which have led to the patient's having been harmed by alcohol. He needs to be taught as much as possible about the stages of alcoholism and faced with his evasions and reluctance to admit his loss of freedom, and his slavery to drink. Discussions can include practice in handling social situations without alcohol, in refusing drinks from 'well-meaning' friends, in improving social confidence and in role-playing of difficult interviews with employers or meetings with estranged relatives. Group discussions with other patients and including recovered alcoholics point up the trenchancy, relevance and yet helpfulness of what is being said.

What is required, if it is done in hospital, is a vigorous and organized regime lasting about a month. Longer periods have not been shown to improve results, and there are disadvantages to them, when the alcoholic who is improving needs, without delay, to resume responsibility for himself in an outside world which includes the ubiquitous availability of alcohol, to rejoin his family if possible, and to get back to work. Indeed there is much to be said for concentrating treatment on outpatient group therapy, held in the community and if possible after usual working hours. In the words of Maggs, admission to a psychiatric hospital can make the condition worse, 'as this procedure very often prevents the on-going resolution of social and personal problems, and the secondary repressive effects of the institution begin to bite as each day passes. To admit a patient having forced out of him a pledge which may be inappropriate or which he is not ready to fulfil is not sound therapy'. Nevertheless, psychiatric admissions are sometimes needed in the hope that relief from total chaos will promote a fresh start, and associated depression or other psychiatric disorder may make admission essential.

The aim is normally to get the patient to commit himself to lasting abstinence, anything less leading to very frequent relapse and loss of control of drinking. It seems rare although perhaps not unknown for alcoholics to be able to return successfully to relaxed social drinking without danger of relapse, and certainly for practical purposes every attempt should be made to get permanent abstinence. Arguments by the patient that he need not give up completely, and will be all right if he sticks to beer, or shandy, are highly suspect of indicating that he is insufficiently alarmed by his drinking problem.

Wavering commitment to abstinence can be bolstered by the use of *drugs imcompatible with alcohol*, such as disulfiram ('antabuse'). The patient takes 200–400 mg daily, and taking a drink is followed by severely unpleasant (and dangerous) flushing, hypotension and possible collapse, as acetaldehyde intoxication releases histamine. The patient has to be warned of the mechanism of the treatment most carefully, and is usually given a small test dose in hospital. The advantage is that the patient commits himself not to drink that day, at a time when he feels confident to make this commitment, and then should be protected, by the real danger alcohol poses to him, from drinking later in the day. The treatment helps those alcoholics who are quite highly determined to abstain, and fails in others, who simply stop taking the tablets. The patient thus retains his freedom to return to drinking.

Alcoholics Anonymous, an organized body of recovered alcoholics, offering meetings and volunteer support including an effective telephone Samaritan service, has a very good record of consistent help to alcoholics. It is increasingly invited to work with the alcoholism service, holding meetings in hospitals and establishing contact with patients and potential members. It works as a supportive peer-group of people who have first-hand knowledge of the problems, with an almost religious philosophy and a crusade to convince its hearers that alcoholism is a disease.

Social rehabilitation. Many alcoholics will have lost most of the social fabric of their lives during their long decline, marriages having been strained and then destroyed, jobs lost, homes abandoned. Progress back to self-respect and repair of relationships requires devoted and resourceful attention from those engaged in helping, especially social workers, whether professional or volunteer. *Hostels* with varying regimes are needed for the first stages after emerging from hospital or coming back into society from skid row, and it is generally agreed that voluntary bodies come into their own here, with fine achievements to their credit.

Supportive psychotherapy to the wives and husbands helps to repair marriages, which repair then gives the patient a far better chance to remain abstinent when supported by his familiar loved ones and not a reject on society's scrap-heap. Alcoholics Anonymous sponsors Al-Anon, a group for the partners of alcoholics to share experiences and support each other.

PROGNOSIS

Alcoholism, once developed, is essentially a continuing danger from a typically relapsing condition. Repeated disappointments must not be allowed to deter the doctor from fresh efforts, and if necessary from rejoicing merely in months or a few years of health and sobriety for the patient before another period of decline. Probably the results vary little in different centres, although recent trends have been to employ short periods of admission, of no more than a month for most patients, followed by an increased emphasis on a full service in the community. Long-term prognosis is much better when the patient is realistic rather than evasive or superficial about his drinking problem at the end of the first period of contact with his professional helpers.

There are some alcoholics whom we fail to persuade to stop destroying themselves, and perhaps a quarter will drink themselves to death. Nevertheless the next time an alcoholic asks for help may be the crucial time, and it behoves us to be ready in case the new effort is genuine, and a man can be saved from sordid ruination.

DRUG ABUSE

DEFINITION

Drugs are substances which are deliberately taken to change the functions of the body or mind. For thousands of years in Western culture alcohol was the principal drug which affected the mind, but now tobacco is equally important. Many of the other substances were originally rare and studied by apothecaries, but the most potent available nowadays have been synthesised in recent times and regarded as the preserve of doctors to prescribe for the ill. So *drug abuse* is excessive use of the drugs outside medical practice, always remembering that doctors might prescribe excessively, and that alcohol and tobacco are in anomalous positions as being by custom beyond medical control. The drugs are regarded as being abused when they are taken for personal pleasure resulting from certain of the mental effects.

Instant pleasure, or at least relief from the present distressing state of mind, is a constant lure, and the drugs are always easy to start but hard to give up: 'Humankind cannot bear very much reality' (T. S. Eliot). The effect wears off, tolerance develops, and the original distress returns, plus early withdrawal feelings of discomfort, so that the easiest thing to do is take more drug, and there is no way out of the vicious circle that is not attended by paying back in discomfort now the relief from distress borrowed by the drug.

Drug dependence develops, defined by the World Health Organization as: 'a state, psychic and sometimes also physical, resulting from the interaction between a living organism and a drug, characterised by behavioural and other responses that always include a compulsion to take the drug on a continuous or periodic basis in order to experience its psychic effects and sometimes to avoid the discomfort of its absence. Tolerance may or may not be present. A person may be dependent on more than one drug'.

LAW

Earlier laws were replaced by the Misuse of Drugs Act 1971 and its Regulations 1973. Irresponsible prescribing can be controlled by supervisory bodies set up by the Home Secretary, and drugs can be prescribed for the maintenance of dependent patients, as opposed to the treatment of disease or injury, only by certain licensed doctors, in the case of opiates and cocaine. The names of these patients must be notified to the Chief Medical Officer at the Home Office. Prescriptions for these drugs and for amphetamines, methaqualone (present in Mandrax) and phenmetrazine must be written in ink, and must be signed and dated in the doctor's handwriting. Flexible powers are provided to allow for new drugs to be controlled rapidly if necessary.

GENERAL FEATURES

Drug abuse and dependence was a small problem in this country until the 1960s. Opium and cocaine dependence had been rare, steady in numbers, and many of the patients were in prescribing professions, of mature years, isolated from each other, and no changes in society were involved. Barbiturates and amphetamines were widely prescribed by family doctors to neurotic patients for long periods, disguising a large but unknown number of drug-dependent but not deteriorating patients, again with no preponderance of young people.

In the 1960s, abuse of opiate drugs, especially heroin, long very common in the United States of America, began to increase in frequency here, especially among the young and unstable, this increase in itself provoking the concern which led to the new legislation from 1967 onwards. Abuse of barbiturates and amphetamines from illicit sources also increased among the young in their teens and early twenties, and fashions developed by which the drugs were often self-administered intravenously. A drug-taking underground subculture developed, the members of which experimented with any drug available, including a variety of hypnotics such as glutethimide (Doriden) and a tablet containing methaqualone (Mandrax), often in mixtures, often intravenously, often sporadically at parties, and sometimes fatally. Alcohol is drunk and cannabis smoked, also at times in irresponsible amounts and combinations, different ways of intoxicating the mind being regarded as almost interchangeable. Teenagers may be able to buy hypnotic tablets on the black market more cheaply than an equivalent dose of alcohol. The availability of, and experiments with, L.S.D. date from the same period.

The people who abuse the modern drugs, yielding to the temptation to experiment dangerously, and to peer pressure in their milieu of friends, are usually already disturbed and unhappy. They tend not to persist in the face of difficulties, but take instant short cuts to relief of tension. Jobs that do not suit are given up in favour of resting and criticizing the bourgeois system, sex is taken in a world of shifting uncommitted relationships, and others' money, property and interests can be subordinated to theirs. Willis concluded of British heroin addicts that they were a series of highly disturbed individuals and 'appeared to have chosen drugs as a form of relief of turbulent feelings against a setting of intrafamilial disturbance with negligible socio-economic deprivation'.

SPECIFIC FEATURES
The following types of drug dependence are defined by W.H.O.

1 Morphine type
2 Barbiturate or alcohol type
3 Amphetamine type
4 Cocaine type
5 Cannabis type
6 Hallucinogenic type

Opiates
People of stable previous personality can sometimes lead successful lives while supplied with regular, even large, doses of these drugs. Where the personality is psychopathic, however, and when the sources are illegal and unscrupulous, the typical decline occurs, into a life of absent interests except the drug and fellow-abusers, and willingness to lie, steal and degrade self or others to get hold of supplies of the drug. A sleepy euphoria is felt by the patient, and small pupils observed by the doctor after each dose, and there is usually a longstanding constipation. Tolerance develops rapidly, and severe addicts may take at least twenty times the therapeutic dose on each occasion. Complications include those of all unskilled and unhygienic intravenous injection, namely cutaneous abscesses, septicaemia and serum hepatitis, with a significant death rate from physical illness, self-neglect, and misadventures with drugs. Clashes with the law lead increasingly into a haphazardly criminal way of life. There is physical dependence, and a withdrawal syndrome with

considerable suffering from restlessness, wakefulness, running nose and eyes, diarrhoea, cramps and pains. In an alert patient with no substitute psychotropic drug, the craving for the drug of addiction then becomes very strong, leading to importunate behaviour.

The important drugs in this group are heroin, morphine, methadone, pethidine, dextromoramide, dipipanone (in 'Diconal') and levorphanol.

Barbiturates

The psychopharmacology of these substances is very similar to alcohol; for example in their actions in depressing higher cerebral function, releasing more primitive behaviour from inhibition, lengthening reaction time and endangering the driving of motor vehicles, in causing drowsiness and slurring of speech in large doses, and in an anticonvulsant action. Marked tolerance develops. The withdrawal syndrome is characterized by severe insomnia, agitation and a danger of grand mal fits. Even after small repeated doses studied experimentally, the E.E.G. is detectably abnormal for at least six weeks, so even in dependent patients maintained on prescriptions, such as those on only a nightly barbiturate tablet for years, complaints of difficulty with sleeping may be well based for at least that length of time during a period of withdrawal. Complications among severe addicts are those of intravenous injection plus accident-proneness when under the influence of the drugs, and death in coma after misadventures with varying doses and combinations of drugs, sometimes including alcohol.

Amphetamine

The drug acts as a cerebral stimulant, arousing vigilance and abolishing sleep and appetite, so that it is popular for prolonging wakefulness and inducing a feeling of being 'high' at parties among people who abuse drugs. Blood pressure rises and the pupils dilate. Tolerance develops, and on large doses a typical mental state is of a paranoid tinge to the restlessly alert perceptions of the patient, and on occasion this becomes a fully fledged paranoid psychosis in clear or almost clear consciousness, closely resembling schizophrenia. On withdrawal, a phase of apathy, drowsiness and depression is typical, with craving for the drug and subterfuges to obtain it. No replacement drug need be prescribed. As well as pure amphetamine derivatives this group of drugs includes phenmetrazine, 'Durophet', 'Drinamyl' and 'Steladex'.

Cocaine

Dependence on this stimulant is now rare and decreasing.

Cannabis

Cannabis, usually smoked as marijuana, hashish, 'weed', 'grass' or 'tea', is a drug with effects of relaxation and euphoria, and changing perceptions, which may lead to actual hallucinations. It has never had much medical use, and has always been legally ostracised far more than was justified by any evidence that it was very harmful. It is widely taken on social occasions, even in the face of severe penalties, and often by people of stable personality, who consider that it should be available for recreation. The true assessment of risk may be that, like alcohol, it can be used in moderation by stable people without undue risk, but not by unstable people with impunity.

L.S.D. (lysergic acid diethylamide)

This synthetic drug, ('acid'), has extremely potent hallucinogenic effects, even in doses of micrograms. It is usually taken sporadically rather than regularly. The vivid and novel perceptual experiences, much discussed and pondered upon in modern writings, and even employed on occasion in psychiatric treatment, are not always found to be enriching ones. States of terror, and long-lasting severe anxiety states afflict some people; the 'bad trip', in which the horrified victim must be protected by his friends or in hospital from desperate or unrealistic actions, being followed by 'flashbacks' and mental self-scrutiny for many months. In the acute stage of distress, chlorpromazine should be prescribed, preferably in large doses and combined with diazepam to secure sedation and drowsiness. Vigorous treatment is advisable, to prevent the chronic syndrome, which when established, is difficult to relieve with psychotherapy and tranquillizers.

TREATMENT

The aim must be to encourage the patients to live without abusing poisonous and dangerous substances, but difficulties arise because the patients often do not really wish to do this. Requests for help may come at times of trouble with the law, ultimatum from spouse or employer, or frightening physical illness. A reluctant patient may then go through the motions of compliance with medical advice only later to default on attendance or discharge himself from a ward after a spell of manipulative attempts to obtain the drug or substitutes for it.

Rapport may need to be established patiently in the clinic, but this takes time, and meanwhile the patient is on drugs and asks for them to be prescribed.

Opiate-dependent patients can be maintained on prescribed drugs by licensed doctors in outpatient clinics; sometimes gradual withdrawal is possible under these circumstances, but more often it will require strict inpatient supervision in a specialized unit and urine tests as checks. A policy of transfer to prescribed methadone has not been very successful, as it creates methadone-dependent patients. Patients who abuse amphetamines and hypnotic drugs may need the latter prescribed in reducing dosage for a short period as part of a regime in which the doctor hopes to help the patient eventually by other means, especially supportive psychotherapy, arranging social work, and liaising with a Probation Officer if there is one who knows the patient. A major attempt to cure barbiturate dependence requires admission and a graded reduction of prescribed doses, because sudden withdrawal carries the danger of grand mal convulsions.

The disturbed personalities of many of the patients have already been mentioned, and a corollary of this is that firm and supportive regimes are needed to try to modify their claims and expectations, and bring about better solutions to life's stresses. For inpatients and outpatients group therapy is employed, with members of staff selected for sympathy combined with skill in this kind of work. The patients are at great risk of relapse when leaving hospital to seek work and a new style of life, and at such times some hostels can provide protection, support and continuing supervisory psycho-therapy, especially, again, if the staff specialize in this work.

PROGNOSIS

Heroin addiction, the most accurately studied, has a considerable death rate, over 1 per cent per year, many failures, and about 20 per cent cures five years later. In general, poor results are obtained with all methods of treatment in the patients with damaged personalities, and the few successes are largely among the more stable individuals. The whole subject is a challenge to the medical profession to do better in future, for the results of punitive measures and prison are certainly no better, while they lack the humane yet practical concern which it is our calling to bring to our patients.

References and Further Reading

Alcohol.
Two indispensable articles are by G. Edwards, 'The meaning and treatment of alcohol dependence', in *Hospital Medicine* 1967, *2*, 272–81, (reprinted in *Contemporary psychiatry* T. Silverstone and B. Barraclough (eds) 1975) and M. M. Glatt, 'Alcoholism', in *British Journal of Hospital Medicine* 1974, *2*, 111–20. The W.H.O. reference is to the Technical Report Series No. 42. DHSS 1973, *Community services for alcoholics and alcoholism* describes official policy. R. Maggs was writing in *British Medical Journal* 1975, 26 July, p. 232. A particularly clear account of the syndrome is by G. Edwards and M. M. Gross, 'Alcohol dependence: provisional description of a clinical syndrome', in *British Medical Journal* 1976, *1*, 1058–61. An excellent book is B. D. Hore's *Alcohol dependence* 1976, London: Butterworths.

Abuse of drugs.
An excellent general survey is T. H. Bewley's 'An introduction to drug dependence', in *British Journal of Hospital Medicine* 1970, *4*, 150–61. J. H. Willis' article is 'Drug dependence: some demographic and psychiatric aspects in U.K. and U.S. Subjects', in *British Journal of Addiction* 1969, *64*, 135–46. A fuller account is the chapter by Bewley and Bewley in *Theory and practice of public health* 5th edn W. Hobson (ed.), 1977, OUP.

Recommended articles on related subjects include, 'Cigarette dependence' by M. A. H. Russell, in *British Medical Journal* 1971, *2*, 330–1 and 393–5; 'Analgesic abuse in psychiatric patients', R. M. Murray, G. C. Timbury and A. L. Linton, *Lancet* 1970, *1*, 1303–5; and 'Pathological gambling' by E. Moran, in *British Journal of Hospital Medicine* 1970, *4*, 59–70, reprinted in *Contemporary psychiatry*, T. Silverstone and B. Barraclough (eds), British journal of psychiatry special publication 1975.

Chapter 15

Mental Handicap

CONCEPT

The names applied have frequently changed, in laudable efforts to reduce stigma and direct attention and services less reluctantly to these unfortunate people. Mental Deficiency became Mental Retardation, and now the best term in general use is Mental Handicap. The terms idiocy, imbecility and feeble-mindedness, originally defined by law, are now not used. The present legal terms are now defined in the Mental Health Act of 1959, which provides for compulsory admission to hospital or for guardianship in the care of a responsible person or authority. The categories are *severe subnormality*: 'a state of arrested or incomplete development of mind which includes subnormality of intelligence and is of such a nature or degree that the patient is incapable of leading an independent life or of guarding himself against serious exploitation or will be so incapable when of an age to do so', and *subnormality*: 'a state of arrested or incomplete development of mind . . . which requires or is susceptible to medical treatment or other special care or training'.

The concept covers all conditions characterized by defective, subnormal mental development from birth or early childhood. The failure of development affects all faculties, intelligence being the most obvious but social competence always being affected at the same time. Handicaps in intellectual and social fields are hardly distinguishable in childhood, because a severely limited rate of development of intelligence limits learning and grasp of the subtleties of social living, and the development of emotional life and of constructive drive are also always affected. Imbalance between the severities of handicap in different faculties certainly occurs, and is important in psychiatry: the problems of a severely subnormal emotionally fairly stable individual are different from those of an equally unintelligent man who is unstable. Commonly intelligence, which can be measured, and social incompetence are both used, whether in legal or clinical definitions.

INCIDENCE

Rates vary in relation to the social competence expected of individuals in the population studied. Approximately 1 per thousand are in hospitals, 3 per thousand need services of some kind, and about 5 per thousand may fulfil the full definitions of social and intellectual incompetence.

AETIOLOGY

1 Subcultural.
2 Pathological (genetic, chromosomal and environmental).
3 Social.

Intelligence is distributed in the population in a way close to the 'normal' distribution, with peak frequency being defined at I.Q. 100 and increasingly high and increasingly low scores becoming rarer the more extreme they are. Below I.Q. 70 are found about 2 per cent of the population, and below I.Q. 45 individuals are rare. Normal individuals free of identifiable pathological condition are in fact unusual among the severely handicapped under I.Q. 45, for the tail of the distribution curve is swollen at the lower end by a population of abnormally developed individuals. The first heading of cause is therefore:

Subcultural Mental Handicap

This concept refers to the fact that the bulk of the mentally handicapped are simply the poorly endowed but not unhealthy individuals at the bottom of the social-intellectual range, just as most very short people are not suffering from diseases of the bones or endocrine glands. The cause is thus mainly the multifactorial inheritance of intelligence and presumably of related endowments. These people tend to be fertile and to be children not of other handicapped people but of the mildly unintelligent, whose even more unintelligent offspring they are. Their siblings on the average are also unintelligent. By contrast the pathologically handicapped are rare, are concentrated among the severe cases, are typically infertile, and are children of parents with a normal spread of levels of intelligence; their siblings also include the range of normally endowed individuals, the patient standing out as the handicapped member of the family.

Pathological Mental Handicap

a) *Specific Hereditary Conditions.* Inborn errors of metabolism transmitted by Mendelian recessive genetic mechanisms account for a number of conditions with severe handicap. Among the rare amino-acidurias *phenylketonuria* is of much the greatest importance. It has an incidence of about 1 in 15,000 in the general population and is usually associated with severe handicap. The patients are often relatively unpigmented fair individuals with overactive behaviour. Adequate arrangements for the welfare of the newborn should nowadays always include testing for phenyl-pyruvic acid in blood or urine. A confirmed positive result needs to be followed by upbringing on a diet restricted in phenylalanine, for there is evidence that when this is started in infancy the degree of subsequent handicap will be greatly reduced.

Lipid-storage disorders include Tay-Sachs' disease in which the patients die in childhood. Among disorders of carbohydrate metabolism *galactosaemia* is the most important, as treatment can be attempted by removing lactose from the diet, after galactose is found in the urine of an infant who is failing to thrive.

Cretinism (congenital hypothyroidism) has been eliminated in its endemic form, which was caused by iodine deficiency in some areas, by iodine supplements in the diet. A sporadic form occurs, however, and may be an inborn error of thyroid metabolism or absence of the gland. Early diagnosis is very difficult, as a typical picture develops only after some months, when the child does not grow, has a yellowish-grey colour, is slow in reaction, apathetic and snuffly. The skin becomes puffy, particularly on the eyelids and lips, hands and feet, and back of the neck; body temperature is subnormal, there are always feeding difficulties, and mental and physical development is stunted. Laboratory proof of the diagnosis is followed by treatment with l-thyroxine by mouth. Some mental function is saved but usually a degree of handicap persists.

Some diseases are inherited as Mendelian dominants, the best known being *tuberous sclerosis* or epiloia. Many abnormalities are found in this condition, including cerebral deformities, adenoma sebaceum and epilepsy. The mental handicap is usually severe, and many patients die young.

Microcephaly, stunting deformity of skull and underlying cerebrum, is common in the severely handicapped and probably includes a variety of conditions which have not yet been clearly distinguished from each other and the causes of which are not known.

b) *Chromosomal Anomalies.* Abnormal configurations of the sex chromosomes as in Klinefelter's syndrome (XXY formula) and the XYY syndrome are probably associated with an increased incidence of mental handicap, but by far the most important condition is *mongolism* or *Down's syndrome.* This condition occurs in about 1 in 700 live births and is always associated with severe mental handicap. The risk rises rapidly with age of the mother; in the 40-year-old mother there is a 1 in 100 risk and after 45 the risk rises to 1 in 25. So typically the mongol is the youngest child in his family. The cause is an anomaly in the amount of chromosome-21 material in the cells of the individual: in most cases this originated by non-separation of the 21-chromosomes in the mother's germ-cell, so that the mongol has trisomy-21 in his cells.

There are many physical abnormalities including the characteristic facial appearance with oblique eyelids, broad nose, flattened head, fissured and enlarged tongue, lax joints, and short stature, small low abnormal ears, broad hands with anomalous creases and maldeveloped little finger, a cleft between the great toe and the rest of the foot, bulging abdomen and various other gastrointestinal and cardiovascular anomalies. Mortality is raised in the early years. Temperamentally mongols tend to be tractable, lively, good-tempered, fond of mimicry, music, rhythm and clowning. They are affectionate, sociable, and usually popular members of the family, despite their gross mental defect.

c) *Environmental Factors.* Many hazards can impair normal development through cerebral damage, the resulting syndrome often bearing no recognizable relation to the damaging cause.

Infections to be considered include rubella, congenital syphilis and toxoplasmosis in utero, and meningitis of viral, acute bacterial or tuberculous origin in early childhood.

Birth injury and anoxia before or during delivery are associated with increased frequency of mental handicap, as is *prematurity* at birth. There is probably a complex mixture of factors here, in that social factors are involved too, for parents in the lower social groups less often seek, and then receive, poorer antenatal care. This in turn predisposes to obstetric complications such as prematurity, anoxia and injury to the foetal head and brain: then development is handicapped by these injuries, but there will also be further hazards from the biochemical immaturity of the premature child: for example neonatal jaundice will be more severe, with the chance of developing kernicterus and further mental retardation. The association of mental handicap with spasticity is also complex, involving an interaction of genetic, prenatal and birth damage. *Head injury* during childhood can also retard development, as can *lead poisoning*. Any of the causes of *hydrocephalus* may act similarly.

Social factors
Although there must be a constitutional capability of the individual, social factors are always involved in the recognition of difficulties resulting from poor endowment. The complex demands of urban life in a crowded city may lead to failure for a man who could manage in the country. Road-sweeping provided simple jobs in town which disappear when machines take over, so that the simple man becomes unemployed, frustrated and a problem. Upper and lower social classes recognise or shelter their feeble brethren differently. Large families are commoner at the bottom of society and the children brought up in them have deprived environments, less of their mother's undivided attention, and probably live in parts of the city with poor obstetric services and worse education. Vicious circles are set up in which handicapped environments hamper the progress of the borderline handicapped who become unable to cope with their lives and produce too many children in poor conditions, and thus continue the cycle into the next generation. Hence the full definition of subcultural mental handicap in Blackie et al (1975): 'a limitation of intelligence based on polygenic inheritance but compounded by severe social and educational disadvantagement so that the majority of these subjects require services (education, social work or medical) at some stage in their lives'.

CLINICAL FEATURES

Congenital abnormalities, anatomical and physiological, are common, especially at low levels, although many individuals with severe handicap appear to be normal physically. Epilepsy is very common.

The severely handicapped are wholly dependent on others for their care and have to be protected against common physical dangers. They cannot be taught to feed themselves, to keep themselves clean, nor can they recognize other people nor communicate with them except in the most primitive way. Their emotional responses reflect this general simplicity. When frustrated they may bite, scratch or kick, but when in happy mood smile and grin.

Those less severely handicapped, while requiring care and protection throughout their lives, can be taught to feed themselves and develop human relationships. Occasionally rote learning develops remarkably in limited fields, but true understanding is missing, with negligible capacity for abstract thought. Often they are happily dependent people who appreciate and respond with simple helpful behaviour to kind, sympathetic handling.

However the immaturity and simplicity of their emotional and intellectual balance may be shown in the response to sexual or aggressive impulsives after (usually late) puberty. Typically instinctual drives are as poorly developed as other aspects of the personality, but sometimes problems arise from failure to control impulses and appreciate the social significance of behaviour. This can lead on occasion to inappropriate sexual advances or demands, heedless aggression and crimes against property. At the same time they can be vulnerable to exploitation by others in prostitution and criminal gangs.

The personality, like that of people of normal intelligence, varies from one individual to another: some are gentle and kindly, others rough, deceitful and vindictive. Like everybody else they display in this not only a constitutional but also a reactive environmental aspect, responding to kindness, being embittered by cruelty, enriched by stimulation, bored by sameness. The capacity of even the best endowed patients, who can be taught a simple trade, depends as much on their character and personality as upon the level of their intelligence.

The handicapped have high rates of psychiatric disorder to contend with as well as the basic limitation of development. The studies of 10-year-old children in the Isle of Wight mentioned on p. 299 showed that one-third of the mentally handicapped were also psychiatrically disturbed. No doubt the causes are to be found in interaction between the malformed brain, and the deprived and rejected lives often experienced by the patients, including in some instances in the past, poor institutions.

In the severely handicapped some patients remain undisturbed, but syndromes of problematic behaviour are frequent. Common are gross hyperkinesis, stereotypies and withdrawal, and a few patients with an intractable condition of severe and multiple disturbances of behaviour damaging to themselves, other people and property.

In the mildly handicapped, the range of psychiatric disorder resembles that in other individuals, A stable person may show a remarkable capacity for adaptation in adult life, provided the stresses and demands are not pressed too far.

Case No. 29

A single woman of twenty-two, was referred by her parents to her General Practitioner, because she had been unable to settle into any kind of training or employment. She had in fact fallen progressively far behind from the age of eight onwards, and although her parents were comfortably off, owning their own retail shop, she had been unable to benefit from the special efforts to educate her which they had made. She had taken no external examinations nor any internal school tests; and had subsided gradually but progressively through each school to which she had been sent, until on leaving school at the age of seventeen, she was two and a half years behind the average. Immediately after school she had expressed a desire to look after young children, and had received a nursery school training through the local authority, which she had failed to complete.

Her parents had then arranged private training in a private institution for young orphan children, but here she had received a very adverse report, because she had tended to lose her temper easily, and occasionally to appear to descend to the children's own level of teasing and spitefulness. At the time of examination she was unemployed.

She presented as a well-dressed but incompetently made-up girl, with an open friendly manner, but very little tolerance or sustained effort, and no insight into her own difficulties. On formal intellectual testing she proved to have an I.Q. of 68, and to be clearly unable to contend either with the standards of abstract comprehension, or the individual responsibilities, of the sort of career which she had stated she desired. Ultimately she was happily settled into a factory making cartons, where her work was repetitive, simple, and obvious.

The handicapped are prone in childhood to profound disturbances of behaviour, largely arising out of their handicaps and the adjustments which they face, and in adult life they may exhibit swings of mood, deliberately grotesque or hysterically exaggerated behaviour or crude versions of schizophrenic symptoms. On the other hand, some may show a remarkable capacity for social adaptation in adult life, provided the stresses and demands are not pressed too far. Nothing need prevent friendship and sexual interests from developing, and recreations such as going to clubs, dancing, crafts, painting and listening to music are as life-enhancing to the handicapped as to anyone else. Marriage can succeed, although some supervision of the welfare of the children will be needed.

DIAGNOSIS

This is based on a close study of the developmental history, examination of the patient, and formal intellectual testing. The I.Q. has in fact turned out to be a good guide to educability although it is less accurate in predicting capacity in adult life. Doctors are often required to give an estimate of the possibility of mental handicap in very young children, either because of anxiety on the part of the parents or in the case of impending adoption. Later, very thorough assessment of educability may be needed at the age of five when school starts.

In infancy it is of value to remember that by twelve weeks a normal child can hold up his head in the prone position, can note and follow with his eyes a dangling toy, can study the movements of his own hands and bear weight on his forearms, and will show a response when spoken to, often making some noise in reply. A handicapped child is likely to do none of these things, and if none of them has been accomplished by the end of twenty weeks it becomes increasingly probable that a significant degree of mental defect underlies this mental incapacity, in the absence of other established disease. The criteria during later childhood will be the same: development must be proceeding at a markedly slow rate for it to become arrested at a low level in the end, and slow development found in all fields tested is strong evidence for mental handicap.

TREATMENT, SERVICES AND TRAINING
(see also Chapter 17)

With good paediatric services, early case-finding will allow treatment of a few biochemical anomalies and cretinism. Coexisting physical handicaps such as epilepsy, poor eyesight, poor hearing, speech defects and weakness of limbs need energetic attention. Otherwise the treatment is essentially the provision of adequate care, education, management and training suited to the capacities and social situation of the individual.

Generally the home is supported as the best place of upbringing, supplementary services being provided for education, training and if necessary professional care away from the family. The policy of promoting community care means that fewer patients are to be admitted to the big old hospitals. Local services need to be organized in specialist teams offering advice and services including residential and occupational help, within easy reach of the patient's home.

In the past many children were virtually abandoned in hospitals, and even in 1978 there remain 4000 among the adults in the long-stay hospitals. Priority is now to be given to alternatives to long-stay institutional care. Some patients still require admission for particularly specialized nursing and medical care, and relief of burdened families may be needed, so that residential placements must be available. Furthermore, parents eventually die, at which point protection has to be arranged by the public service.

Education for all children has been the responsibility of the education service since 1971. Children in the community above approximately I.Q. 50 can usually be educated in schools for the educationally subnormal to the age of 16 (80,000 mildly and 33,000 severely affected children in special schools), on a day or residential basis, those more severely handicapped receiving training in dressing, personal cleanliness, habits of work, clear speech and good behaviour to others. Day hospitals with nursing for the incontinent may provide relief for the parents and bring about some progress in the children who are barely educable.

Adolescents and adults attend training centres from home or residential hostels to continue training in work and social skills, and mixing with the opposite sex. Typical problems at the time of adolescence are frustration at inability to find a job, families becoming intolerant of the fully grown but mentally handicapped member, vulnerability to sexual exploitation in girls, and delinquency in boys. Some individuals will be able to progress to work in sheltered workshops or even to unskilled jobs. Social clubs under supervision can help to counteract the frustration and humiliation resulting from knowledge of one's social awkwardness and inexperience.

The parents need support and information as much as their children need care and training. Counselling should include knowledge of the local services, genetic counselling advice, discussions of family planning, offers of financial help and free laundry to those coping with the incontinent, and the availability of offers to admit the patient for an occasional relief period to allow for family holidays or respite in times of crisis. The voluntary societies such as the National Society for Mentally Handicapped Children also help parents, not least by arranging contacts and mutual support groups.

PREVENTION

In pathological defect separate projects against conditions with known and treatable causes can have important results, and genetic counselling may be expected to reduce the frequency of some conditions. Reducing the fertility of the handicapped themselves, often suggested, would not contribute very greatly to preventing the condition even if it were humanely promoted, for only about a tenth of the mildly handicapped are in fact offspring of the handicapped of the previous generation. The only promising approach involves reducing the high fertility of the unskilled: when a child is found to be handicapped a major and intense effort to deliver birth control advice to the parents might reduce the number of further siblings in that family and this would, if an effective policy, reduce the pool of subcultural mental handicap in the next generation. At the same time there is much to be said for educational priority being given to these families and their children, so that they may be trained to manage marginally better, to seek full obstetric care, to bear only small families and to arrange, so far as they are innately capable, stimulating environments for their children.

References and Further Reading

There are excellent textbooks on the subject, such as *Mental retardation*, 2nd edn, by R. F. Tredgold and K. Soddy, 1970, Aberdeen University Press. Mongolism is reviewed by C. Scully in *British Journal of Hospital Medicine*, July 1973, and subcultural mental defect by J. Blackie et al. in *British Journal of Psychiatry* 1975, *127*, 535–9. Public policy is described in *Better services for the mentally handicapped*, Cmnd 4683, H.M.S.O. 1971, and family life vividly in '*Bernard – bringing up our mongol son*', by John and Eileen Wilkes, 1974, Routledge and Kegan Paul.

In a rapidly changing field the most modern approaches will be found in *New perspectives in mental handicap* by A. Forrest et al., Edinburgh, Churchill Livingstone 1973; the National Development Group for the Mentally Handicapped report *Day services for mentally handicapped adults* (1977) H.M.S.O.; Casework is described well in *The mentally subnormal – social work approaches*, by M. Adams and H. Lovejoy, 2nd ed. London, Heinemann, 1972; *Mental handicap* by B. Kirman and J. Bicknell (eds) London, Churchill Livingstone 1975, and *Mental deficiency: the changing outlook* by A. M. Clarke and A. D. B. Clarke (eds), London, Methuen 1974.

Chapter 16

Psychiatric Emergencies

This chapter deals with psychiatric emergencies as they may present to the general practitioner, general surgeon, physician or obstetrician. Most clinical situations are described in their respective chapters, but some additional account of important ones is given here.

ATTEMPTED SUICIDE

INTRODUCTION

This is a most important emergency, which may confront any doctor at any time.

It happens whenever a dangerously disturbed patient has attempted, for example, to throw himself out of the window, or into a river, or under a bus, and has been prevented at the last moment from coming to serious harm. Increasingly in the last twenty years it happens by self-inflicted cutting of the wrist and especially after ingestion of an overdose of drugs, commonly with alcohol as well.

The incidence of self-poisoning has been rising sharply, so that these cases are now a major type of admission to medical wards. Social trends in the kind of behaviour resorted to in situations of stress are involved, and many of the incidents mimic attempted suicide rather than being true examples of it. Nevertheless, even putting aside the unhappiness and desperation of the patient at the time and his physical danger, they are hazardous situations for the future, in at least two ways. First, a patient who has attempted suicide, or acted in a similar fashion, has a considerably raised chance of death by suicide in succeeding years, and second, the degree of this risk cannot be estimated from the seriousness of the poisoning or the depth of the cuts on the wrist in the original incident.

Attempts at suicide are commoner in the young than the old, and in women than in men. They are frequently associated with emotionally unstable personalities, although they also occur in dangerous situations in seriously ill patients.

DIFFERENTIAL DIAGNOSIS

In practice four conditions are likely to be responsible for this situation. They are

1 Hysterical states, and situations involving emotional pressure on others in the patient's entourage – e.g. to secure some action that the patient wants, or to make someone feel guilty for having made the patient so desperate.
2 Depressive states.
3 Schizophrenic illnesses.
4 Patients under the influence of alcohol or drugs (and who may of course be in the situations 1, 2, and 3 above).

MANAGEMENT

The doctor's first essential duty is to make quite sure that the potential capacity for inflicting serious harm no longer exists (no concealed razor blades, pills, etc.). Next, if a substantial amount of toxic substance has been involved, urgent admission may be needed to a medical unit for the observation and treatment of poisoning. The principles of the medical treatment of poisoning will not be discussed further here except to underline the dangerous unpredictability of salicylate poisoning in the deceptively alert patient, and to point out the complex pharmacology and danger of fatal collapse found after the ingestion of several groups of drugs often available to psychiatric patients, including the tricyclic antidepressants, the mono-amine oxidase inhibitors and the barbiturates.

Patients admitted to hospital for the treatment of acute poisoning must always be under the care of the medical department, for reasons of safety, with advice from the psychiatrists being offered to the physicians on the subsequent psychiatric care of the patient.

If the doctor does not decide that there is a danger of poisoning from drugs already taken, he still has to judge whether the patient intends to renew the attempt in the immediate future. If in his judgment the patient does so intend, then admission to hospital may need to be insisted upon to save the patient's life, and on rare occasions this may even need to be done with an Order for Observation under Section 25 of the Mental Health Act (see Chapter 18). It is ethically not only justifiable but imperative to act in this way when there is danger and the likelihood of mental illness having impaired the patient's ability to make decisions about his life. Only in this way can irreversible desperate actions be prevented in the short run, with the possibility of helping the patient and treating curable illnesses in hospital. Later his freedom to do what he wishes with his own life is restored when he leaves.

If on the other hand the doctor is satisfied that there is no immediate danger of a repetition of the attempt, and the patient is otherwise not seriously harmed, then urgent attempts to gain immediate admission to hospital are unnecessary; and may even lead to the emergence of panic on all sides, particularly among the relatives. The immediate requirements of the situation are:

1 Put such patients to bed, but not in order to leave them alone.
2 Be prepared to spend enough time with them, at least to learn from them in their own way what has been going on and why they acted as they did.
3 Provided that the situation was not one of overdosage of drug or alcohol, give a substantial but safe sedative for that night, and see the following morning. For example, nitrazepam 10–15 mg, chlorpromazine 100–200 mg, or possibly pentobarbitone 100–300 mg, according to the size and vigour of the patient.

Thereafter the indications for admission to hospital, or further treatment at home or through an outpatient department, can be considered when the immediate crisis has passed, in the light of the diagnosis and the patient's condition (see case No. 15).

GENERAL CONSIDERATIONS

In all cases of attempted suicide, and even of irresponsibly dangerous acts simulating it, once the immediate crisis has been dealt with by whatever medical or surgical means are appropriate, it must be remembered that the essence of the situation is that a human being has risked or decided to choose death as the only solution to an overwhelming threat or disaster. It is therefore the doctor's duty to discover the nature of this threat or disaster, and the ways in which it can be made in some way manageable or endurable for the patient. In hysterical suicidal attempts, this may be simply a matter of personal or environmental acceptance, understanding, and help. In cases of depression, or schizophrenia, it will call for at least a limited period of admission to hospital. In all cases the doctor must act towards the patient as friend and saviour, rather than as pure technician, or agent of curative or legal processes.

ACUTE HYSTERICAL STATES

These are of two kinds:

1. Hysterical collapse.
2. Hysterical acting out.

They can occur in the absence of present discoverable structural illness of any kind, but they are always an indication that a human being in distress has found no better solution than a partial surrender of mental and emotional integrity. Their motivation is always partly unconscious, but frequently they symbolize some kind of escape, relief, or possible solution which the patient cannot achieve in any other way.

Hysterical Collapse

This, as we have seen, may be simply the sudden *loss of a previously normal faculty*, such as power or sensation in one or more limbs, loss of vision, loss of speech, loss of hearing, loss of consciousness, or loss of previously normal memory. The key to diagnosis is that the patient has been previously in a situation of environmental stress or threat and that on examination there is no discoverable evidence of damage or disease in the central nervous system or elsewhere. The patient may be co-operative, reluctant, or inaccessible. Immediate treatment should rest on three essential steps:

(1) Put the patient to bed.

(2) See the patient alone; and give him the opportunity of communicating whatever he can about the nature of his predicament, without a sense of hurry, impatience, or hostile criticism.
Acceptance, and an air of compassionate understanding, will
not only represent the reasonable and human approach, but
will often set the stage for solving the problem.

(3) If necessary, give an adequate nocturnal sedative (see last
section of this chapter) and revisit the next morning.

Then, if the situation does not seem to be clear or under control,
a psychiatric opinion as a relative emergency is justified. Alternatively, a psychiatric consultation at a convenient time can be
arranged in the light of what has emerged in the immediate handling
of the case.

Hysterical Acting Out

This differs from hysterical collapse in that the patient may be
creating a scene, or behaving in a way likely to cause alarm and
despondency in others (he is thought to be 'acting out' his emotional
problems on those around him, rather than suffering them within
himself). The doctor's immediate decision is whether or not any
means other than seeing the patient alone, which is often effective
in itself, will be necessary to control the situation. If further
measures are necessary, they amount simply to quietening the
patient temporarily by appropriate sedatives. (See above, but the
chlorpromazine can also be given intramuscularly, and diazepam
or barbiturates can be given, also intramuscularly, or slowly by
the intravenous route).

The patient can be interviewed later, as in the preceding section,
either while the drug is taking effect, or after it has worn off.
Interviews with the other people involved will also be essential
for a full understanding of the situation, as described in Chapter 9.

AGGRESSIVE BEHAVIOUR

Doctors are often called to episodes of aggressive behaviour, with
attacks on property or people, whether in the home, where a
number of frightened people are found surrounding and controlling
the fighting man, or in Casualty departments, whither the police
have brought him.

The *differential diagnosis* includes:

1. *Acute paranoid schizophrenic states*, in which a patient with hallucinatory voices and delusions of persecution becomes increasingly angry, impulsive and out of touch with reason and reality. He may start to fight back against the fancied agents of the persecution which he is sure he suffers.

2. *States of manic or catatonic excitement.* In mania the patient is rarely dangerous to other people except when his overactivity has been inadvisedly restrained and frustrated. The treatment is as described in Chapter 7. Catatonic states escalate without external provocation – this is described more fully below.

3. *Organic states* may limit impulse control at the same time as impairing grasp of the external world so that the confused patient fights those around who were trying to help deal with him. *Epilepsy* is particularly associated with severe mood swings, short temper, confusion and severe violence once control is lost. In epileptic aggressive emergencies, a number of helpers may be needed, together with medication with substantial doses of diazepam or barbiturates.

4. *Drugs and alcohol* further impair control of aggression in the above states, and frequently complicate social crises involving non-psychotic aggression, mentioned below. As well as drunkenness and similar states induced by other cerebrally depressant drugs, the disturbed behaviour may concern stimulant drugs of the amphetamine type. Drunkenness in itself is not a psychiatric emergency, and if the subject's physical condition is safe from the point of view of alcohol poisoning, recent head injury and other unrecognized medical conditions, and if associated mental illness is not present, it is not necessary for the doctor to take full responsibility for the outcome. Sobering-up at the scene of consultation, or leaving the matter to the police, may be appropriate measures.

5. Many emergencies are concerned not with any of the above but with aggressive behaviour which has occurred after *loss of temper* in a normal person or someone with long-standing traits of impulsive and fearsome aggressiveness (*'psychopathic aggression'*). Police, doctor, or both may be called, and the doctor may find a scene of destruction and a struggling patient restrained by several men. The aim will be to remove the restraint in conditions of safety, reducing the number of people present as it becomes evident that patient and doctor are now safe with each other. If the subsequent

interview does not reveal evidence of mental illness, medical treatment may not be required, or indeed desirable. There are important reasons for reluctance to admit patients to psychiatric units for psychopathic violence: the patient is labelled as ill and not responsible for his behaviour; it starts a pattern of resort to medical care and hospital at times of what are really violent tempers; the psychiatric service may have no relevant treatment the following day; and the treatment of other patients may be disrupted.

Nevertheless, diagnosis is hard to establish at the time and there are occasions when a psychiatric admission of a sedated patient may be unavoidable. More usually, the aim should be for supervised calming down at home, or intervention by the police.

ACUTE PSYCHOTIC DISTURBANCES

Psychiatric emergencies, for example arising in the course of intercurrent medical or surgical illness, and presenting usually as progressive loss of contact between the patient and his environment, with varying degrees of clouding of consciousness and associated excitement, stupor or panic, can be divided into two main groups:

1. Delirium (acute confusional states), and
2. Acute episodes of functional psychosis.

Delirium (Acute Confusional States)

In the acute form these are common emergencies in hospital wards and at home, when patients are ill and cerebral function is affected, sometimes the impairment caused by the original illness being unintentionally made worse by drugs and other forms of treatment. The subject is described fully in Chapter 5.

Acute Episodes of Functional Psychosis

These acute psychotic episodes are really sudden explosions of the classical forms of mental illness, occurring in people constitutionally liable to such illness, and released in this instance by environmental stress, or by medical or surgical crises. They comprise essentially:

(1) Acute schizophrenic episodes ⎫
(2) Acute depressive episodes   ⎬ including puerperal episodes
(3) Acute mania   ⎭ of these conditions

These will be dealt with collectively here, although acute depressive and catatonic schizophrenic episodes will require further specific consideration below. The differential diagnosis of acute episodes of functional psychosis from toxic confusional states can usually be made relatively easily on three grounds:

1 the history, both previous, personal and medical history, and the family history, in which evidence of the latent psychosis may be apparent.
2 the absence of the toxic confusional physiological state, and particularly of the six features listed in Chapter 5 (clouding of consciousness, failure of attention, concentration and judgment, disorientation, emotional lability, and hallucinations and misinterpretations).
3 the clinical picture itself, which it may nevertheless take an experienced eye to differentiate in a particular case.

In general, acute psychotic episodes tend to last longer than toxic confusional states, involving as they do a more profound disturbance of basic personality, and they tend to occur in a setting nearer to the normal physiological equilibrium than that seen in acute toxic deliria.

TREATMENT OF ACUTE PSYCHOTIC EMERGENCIES IN GENERAL

The first essential in treatment is to remember that the patient is frightened, estranged, and for this reason often inaccessible and, perhaps, frankly hostile to the normal somewhat detached clinical approach. No matter how disturbing the patient's conduct may be to others, it is he himself who suffers and is disturbed the most of all. And it is to him primarily that the doctor's and nurse's obligation to understand, accept, and relieve, must be fulfilled. Bearing in mind these essential considerations, whose importance cannot be over-emphasized, the following general principles then clearly emerge:

1 *Nursing*: this is as described in Chapter 5 under Toxic Confusional States.

2 *Specific Treatment of Toxic Confusional States* as described in Chapter 5. Existing treatment is reviewed to detect and treat underlying causes. A common cause in emergencies in hospital is an acute withdrawal syndrome in a patient who is not realized to be a habitual consumer of large amounts of barbiturates or alcohol. A full list of causes is given in Chapter 5.

Vitamins and sedation will be required. Diazepam in doses commonly up to 100 mg daily and sometimes more, or chlormethiazole in repeated doses of 0·5 to 1·0 g, are often the drugs of choice, especially in alcohol withdrawal states, but also for toxic confusional states due to other causes. Both drugs can be given orally or intravenously. Both are sedative and mildly hypnotic, anticonvulsant, weakly muscle-relaxant, and safe in large doses. Chlormethiazole has a side effect of causing nasal and bronchial irritation and should not be given to patients with established respiratory difficulty. These drugs can be given in diminishing doses over one to two weeks, as the patient recovers.

Haloperidol is the most useful drug for ˙controlling many of these emergencies. It can be given in doses of 5 to 20 mg intramuscularly in emergency. When haloperidol is given, dyskinetic symptoms, distressing to the patient, sometimes occur, and can be treated by the administration of an anti-parkinsonian drug such as procyclidine hydrochloride (kemadrin) 10 mg intramuscularly or in divided doses by mouth.

3 *Specific treatment of acute psychotic reactions* which are not basically toxic, confusional or delirious in origin.

The same general principles as set out in 1 above apply with equal cogency. The specific medicinal treatment will however lean more upon chlorpromazine which may be given intramuscularly in doses up to 100 mg every four to six hours, or haloperidol in the doses already described.

The management of acute episodes of functional psychosis is otherwise very similar to that of toxic confusional states, and in terms of the human and indeed the professional obligations of those caring for the patient, they are identical. In this connection some final general principles require emphasis.

FINAL GENERAL PRINCIPLES

1 Remember that confusional states are not uncommon, but often avoidable.

2 Think ahead and think early. (The sick patient who is becoming restless at 6 p.m. will often, if untreated, have become wildly disturbed and violently excited by 2 a.m.).

3 Accept the management of these cases as part of every doctor's and every nurse's job: not as a disgraceful catastrophe for which responsibility can be shelved or shoved elsewhere. Remember that among other things doctors and nurses need to stand in patients' eyes as pillars of confidence, acceptance, charity in the true sense, and abiding care. No self-respecting doctor or nurse would shrink from a stinking wound or a sudden haematemesis; still less should they dissociate themselves from the proper care of the acutely disturbed and critically ill patient. As in so many therapeutic techniques, success or failure is ultimately determined by intelligent imaginative anticipation, and the fundamental attitude of mind in approaching the problem.

SPECIAL INSTANCES OF ACUTE PSYCHOTIC STATES

Acute paranoid and catatonic states

a) rapidly progressive excitement, to the point of frenzy.
b) involving rapidly progressive inaccessibility to the point of stupor.

These require immediate and effective action. This is simple:
   Clear the surroundings of the patient of all except one or two sensible trusted friends.
   If the patient is becoming wildly excited, hostile, suspicious or accusatory, talk to him gently, with kindness, and in an obviously unafraid fashion. Find out if possible *what seems to him* to be happening. Prepare to sedate him by announced, explained, and unthreatening administration of intramuscular chlorpromazine up to 100 mg or haloperidol 20 mg. If a responsible assistant is available to steady the arm, these drugs can be given intravenously, or merciful sleep may be obtained by giving intravenous sodium amylobarbitone 0·5 g.
   This treatment will suffice for any stage of excitement or

impulsive frenzy; while a rapid onset of inaccessibility leading to stupor will often respond to a combination of intravenous sodium amylobarbitone, and personal contact. Even if it does not, the indications for removal to hospital are absolute, and the procedure is easy, in the light of the patient's general condition.

Terrified agitated depression
This will be characterized by a combination of frantic despair, inconsolable grief and apprehension, and a general level of agitation and inaccessibility which will have proved exceedingly alarming to all concerned with the patient. The patient himself may well have been sleepless, dehydrated, and have taken little or no food, for days. Such patients require prompt admission to hospital as emergencies; but meanwhile the immediate treatment must be directed towards restoring the patient's psychological and physiological equilibrium by:

a) Gaining personal contact and rapport, so far as possible, with a simple but insistently reassuring attitude.
b) Administering diazepam 10 to 20 mg orally or intramuscularly, and intravenous vitamin B if nutrition is seriously affected.
c) If it proves impossible to get the patient into hospital before nightfall, nocturnal sedation should be administered in substantial dose (nitrazepam 15 mg, chloral 2·0–3·0 g, chlorpromazine 150 mg or pentobarbitone 200–300 mg).

Depressive stupor
Here the patient will have passed through a phase of absolute despair into profound inertia, and finally will have become stuporose and inaccessible. The eyes are usually open, sometimes tear-laden, usually unblinking for long periods; the face grave and ashen; pulse slow and full, posture bowed and motionless.

Treatment does not differ from that of agitated depression except that it is obviously unnecessary to give sedatives, although intravenous sodium amylobarbitone given slowly will often produce temporary accessibility. Press oral fluids, but if the patient is seriously dehydrated and cannot be persuaded to drink, parenteral or intragastric fluids may be given. This is very rarely necessary, as almost all patients will drink if enough patience and care are devoted to persuading them; and anyway their admission to hospital should not be delayed for complicated resuscitative measures elsewhere.

The immediate treatment in hospital for depressive stupor may involve the administration of electrical treatment under anaesthetic, so it is advisable always to inform the hospital if the patient has in fact taken a substantial amount of food or liquid before admission.

CONCLUSION

One of the most striking discoveries which the doctor working for the first time in an acute psychiatric admission unit may expect to make, is that virtually all psychiatric emergencies, properly handled, tend to subside within forty-eight hours. The underlying lessons from this are that the immediate calmness, confidence, kindness and resource of the doctor who first sees the patient, initiates treatment and arranges admission starts him far along the road to recovery, and that the arrival from turmoil outside into safe professional surroundings further reduces many states of great disturbance, even before more specific treatment is embarked upon. Psychiatric emergencies often present as alarming and challenging crises: but the personal attitude of the physician is always invaluable and often decisive in their management and outcome; and the simple and human resources outlined in this chapter will frequently prove entirely effective in their immediate control.

Further Reading

Psychiatric emergencies, edited by R. A. Glick *et al.* 1976, Grune & Stratton, is set in American casualty departments, but describes the clinical situations particularly well and has many useful suggestions on interviewing.

Chapter 17

Policy, Planning and Services

POST-WAR CHANGES

The year 1945 saw the psychiatric services still in the traditional pattern. What little provision there was, existed overwhelmingly as the huge county mental hospitals, usually outside the towns, and in fact often in remote country at the end of a Sunday afternoon bus service for visitors. For most patients the admission procedure was formidable and terrifying, and even the voluntary patients yielded up everything to the gaunt institution while they were in it. There were very small university psychiatric departments, exiguous outpatient clinics, hardly any Day Hospitals; a little private practice.

Many of the roots of the modern changes in the psychiatric services go back to the turbulent times of 1945 and after, and some of them even to the Army Hospitals. For it was in this Service that the first experiments in group therapy and therapeutic community methods were tried in whole wards of psychiatric patients. Interest in how patients' behaviour was affected by the morale of the wards and how they were run, spread to the mental hospitals, where already there was a mood of optimism about treating severe depression and schizophrenia with the recently introduced electrical treatment.

Experiments followed, greatly daring, with unlocking the doors of 'closed' wards. Dire predictions of disaster were proved untrue; patients responded to kindness with gratitude; there were no outbreaks of violence and disorder. Bold spirits opened the doors of yet more highly disturbed wards, the two sexes were allowed to mix, long-forgotten visitors were encouraged to come again, clothing was improved, wards decorated and the patients given wardrobes and their own toilet accessories. All the moves towards making the asylums more like hospitals and less like prisons were followed by improvements not only in the morale of staff and patients, but also in the actual health of the patients.

Then in 1954 an extraordinary thing happened: the ever-rising number of patients in the mental hospitals (half the total beds in the country) reached a peak after over a hundred years, and the next year it fell. The drop in numbers has continued ever since, although it is gently flattening out. The causes of this revolutionary and completely unexpected change have been much discussed. The above-mentioned improvements in the mental hospitals, which were gaining momentum from 1945 onwards, were doubtless important, but it cannot be ignored that 1953 and 1954 saw the introduction of the first effective treatment for the major illness of the hospitals, namely schizophrenia. Probably the two factors acted in combination, for chlorpromazine obtains poor results in poor hospitals, and the new open door policy could not have gone so far without the confidence engendered by the improvement of the highly disturbed schizophrenic patients when they were given the new drug.

1959 MENTAL HEALTH ACT AND 1960 HOSPITAL PLAN

As the patients improved and were discharged home, enthusiasm for a new era in psychiatry grew. Day Hospitals and outpatient clinics opened, and efforts were made to get treatment to the patients early in their illness. The institutions not only of bricks and mortar but of the law were felt to be from an out-of-date era and in need of change. In 1959 all the legislation relating to mental disorder was codified in a new Mental Health Act. This is described more fully in the next chapter, but it can be emphasized here that it encouraged admission of less seriously ill patients without legal formalities, and promoted care in the community. In 1960 the first Hospital Plan appeared, announcing as national policy that future psychiatric units would be in general hospitals, and not in isolation, and that mental hospitals would eventually be able to close.

PROGRESS

The number of mentally ill in hospital has continued to fall, from 154,000 in England in 1954 to two-thirds of that figure in 1973. The wards are less crowded and in fact the mental hospitals are greatly improved in every way. The units in general hospitals are still few, however, accounting in 1973 for only 23 per cent of psychiatric admissions. In mental handicap there has been no comparable revolution in treatment, and around 50,000 patients remain in institutions, with a rising proportion of them being severely disabled or elderly.

But enthusiasm for discharge to the community has often run ahead of provision in the community for the still partially handicapped patients sent home, and the provision of hostels and supportive social work, paid for out of local authority taxation, has in many areas remained very poor. Many of the vagrants in the city streets, and many of the inmates of prisons who have committed repeated but petty crimes, are former patients of mental hospitals, discharged and thereafter neglected. The open door policy became, in cynically ironic phrase, the 'revolving door policy'. Re-admissions rose, and the typical length of stay of the mentally ill patient in hospital is now from two to six weeks.

Does the community care? When support, treatment and acceptance by the staff of the public service are seen to be lacking, the tolerance of families, friends and neighbours is strained to the utmost, and when they are exhausted and exasperated, it is the patient who suffers. If the patient being sent home is still handicapped, the doctors and nurses who send him should have to justify their decision to transfer the patient from professional to amateur care, however devoted it may sometimes be, and however crippling and however much to be avoided are the effects of long-term institutionalization in mental hospital.

REORGANIZATION OF SOCIAL SERVICES

Action on the Seebohm report of 1970 created large united departments of Social Services, with a policy that discouraged the specialization of knowledge by different members of the staff. A major disadvantage has been the loss and waste of skill with the mentally ill and handicapped which had been slowly acquired by experienced specialists in the earlier system. Most of the experienced were promoted to administrative posts at the time of reorganization, and there has been very little psychiatric training for student social workers anywhere. Fortunately this is to some extent being seen now as a case of the pendulum swinging too far, and specialization in skill and sensitivity with the mentally ill is again being encouraged in some quarters, although only to a disappointing extent.

PRESENT POLICIES

The emphasis away from hospitals towards care in the community continues, and mental hospitals and mental handicap hospitals are expected to be needed very much less in future. All new psychiatric units for the mentally ill are to be planned as departments of district general hospitals, and since the reorganization of the National Health Service in 1974, the principal unit in which the services are managed is the District, a typical size of which is a town of 250,000 population. Such a town should have plans for 125 beds for admitting the mentally ill, and the Day treatment departments need about 160 places, most of them for the inpatients but some for day patients. A small unit will be used for the joint assessment of illnesses in the elderly, by psychiatrists and geriatricians, and the care of senile and arteriosclerotic dementia will need another 80–100 beds, perhaps in more local small community hospitals, as well as Day units and transport services.

Specialized units serving larger areas, and sometimes on separate sites or at the old mental hospitals, will be provided for children and adolescents, for alcoholics and drug addicts, and secure units for a small number of patients who at present cannot be cared for in open mental hospitals yet should not have to go to Broadmoor Hospital.

The local authorities are expected by the policy of the Department of Health and Social Security to aim to provide some 150 places for the mentally ill in Day Centres for shelter, occupation and rehabilitation for this hypothetical 250,000 population, as well as a residential hostel for rehabilitation with 10–15 places and longer-stay accommodation for four times as many. Extensive provision of case-work by social workers is also envisaged, but much closer liaison and more money than that found up till now will be needed if this standard of community care is to be realized.

In the mental hospitals, the chronic schizophrenics of yesteryear can in many cases not be looked after anywhere else without cruelty, because in the process of the disease burning out the patient has had to make the hospital his home. These patients die year by year and are not replaced by as many younger patients needing long-term asylum. So the hospitals will continue to get smaller, although very slowly, and there are problems over how to save morale and recruit good staff during the coming years. There will be a need for imaginative schemes integrating the staff and resources of the acute and chronic hospitals in a joint service, and some of the specialized units mentioned above, as well as some rehabilitative tasks, are eminently suitable for keeping on mental hospital sites.

For mental handicap the policy is to allow for the experimental development of small units in various sites, plus networks of supporting services for patients living at home, including especially transport to Day Centres. No more large remote institutions will be built. The policy states that the requirements for a quarter-million population will be of the order of 150 places for the education of severely handicapped children, 370 for the occupation and training of adults in the community, some 200 places in a variety of forms of residential accommodation in the community, and hospital facilities for about 50 children and 160 adults.

There is increasing emphasis on *multidisciplinary team work*, by which is meant all the professional workers such as doctor, nurse, occupational therapist, clinical psychologist and social worker, pooling ideas and to some extent sharing responsibility in the decisions. In the family practitioner's service, he will be the leader of the team with ultimate responsibility for decisions involving the patient's health, and in the specialist therapeutic team the official policy is that 'the consultant psychiatrist normally has responsibility for ensuring that the needs and progress of each patient are regularly reviewed and that other members of the team are involved in these reviews'.

NEW DEVELOPMENTS

Psychiatric nurses have been appointed to posts in which their work is primarily in the community, not even in outpatient clinics, but in the patients' houses, succouring and treating them and also advising and helping families (as described for example in the section on treatment of schizophrenia in the community in Chapter 6), and acting as personal links with the family doctor and the more formal facilities of the clinic, Day Hospital and admission unit. A training course in behavioural psychotherapy for nurses, teaching them to be highly skilled, and independent, has been highly successful and will doubtless be emulated widely.

Clinical psychologists have changed their role as rapidly as their numbers have increased, and now see a main part of their job as being work in a variety of forms of counselling and psychotherapy, many of them scarcely or not at all indebted to medical traditions for their development. The psychologists will be graduates in general psychology, after which there is a two or three year specialized training in clinical work, and the first work with patients is supervised by seniors in the same profession. The clinical psychologist is therefore nowadays independent in his professional standing, with a wide variety of skills to offer the patients referred to him.

Participation by the clinical professions in the planning of their local services is part of the method of the reorganized N.H.S. by means of the Health Care Planning Teams, usually for Mental Illness and Mental Handicap. These are small groups, with a psychiatrist and family practitioner among the members, and they meet to consider the desirable future service for the District, an area which is familiar to them at work and small enough to allow different local styles of service to be suggested and developed on the basis of local enthusiasm.

After decades of neglect, in which money has all too often gone to prestigious expensive projects in the physical specialities, there is much to be done.

References and Further Reading

The topics of this chapter are covered more fully by a number of authors in *Policy for action – a symposium on the planning of a comprehensive district psychiatric service*, R. H. Cawley (ed.) 1973, Nuffield Provincial Hospitals Trust, London, Oxford University Press. The recent statements of official policy are *Better services for the mentally handicapped* 1971, Cmnd 4683, London H.M.S.O., and *Better services for the mentally ill* 1975, Cmnd 6233, London, H.M.S.O. which are excellent essays on their subjects.

Chapter 18

Psychiatry and the Law

In all aspects of the relationship between psychiatry and the law, it is the law which calls the tune. The law defines the basis of the relationship, and by definition is the final arbiter in all interpretations of medico-legal problems. Four fundamental legal principles underlie the whole of forensic psychiatry, and from the standpoint of justice they are unexceptionable. They are:

A sane man is assumed to be wholly responsible for his actions and to intend their consequences.

Just as innocence must be presumed while guilt has to be proved, so equally must sanity be presumed, and insanity proved to the satisfaction of a judge and jury in Crown Court, before it can be legally accepted.

Criminal responsibility is essentially an affair of mind as well as body, of intention as well as action (although some crimes are exceptions to this rule). This is a principle which has been enshrined in English law for nearly 800 years: it is embodied in the famous legal tag *'Actus non facit reum nisi mens sit rea'*. ('There cannot be a guilty act unless there is a guilty mind'.)

No man may be deprived of liberty indefinitely, or of the privilege of managing his own affairs, on purely medical grounds: such deprivation even if necessitated in a patient's own interests and entirely by his unsoundness of mind, may be recommended, and in emergency undertaken by a doctor; but must always be ratified by the decision of the duly appointed and legally authorized representative body or individual. This will be, in the case of deprivation of liberty, a mental welfare officer (social worker) of the local authority, a judge or tribunal, and in the case of management of property, by the Court of Protection, as described below.

These principles form the basis of all laws concerned with mental illness, now consolidated in the Mental Health Act of 1959; they are held also throughout the whole body of common law, whenever this has to do with the assessment of a person's mental state.

In practice the legal implications of psychiatry may be summarized under six headings:

1. Civil responsibility.
2. Criminal responsibility.
3. The Mental Health Act and individual liberty.
4. Psychiatric forms of disposal for mentally abnormal offenders.
5. Management of property.
6. Problem of consent to medical treatment.

Civil Responsibility

Medical opinion as to an individual's state of mind may be required in law to assist in deciding

(1) whether he is competent to give evidence
(2) whether he is competent to enter into a civil contract: this includes marriage as well as contracts of a commercial kind
(3) whether he is competent to recognize and fulfil his normal legal obligations, independently of contract. An infringement or failure to respect the general rights of others, independently of contract, is known as tort; the law of torts, and their relationship to unsoundness of mind, is one of the most complicated aspects of English jurisprudence.
(4) whether he is competent to make a valid will. Here specific examination is required, to test that the patient knows what living relatives he has and can discuss their respective claims, has no abnormal mental state which would be relevant (such as delusions of persecution by one relative), and can remember the will once it has been completed.

In every case the doctor must be guided by his knowledge of the patient, by his recognition of the nature of the disturbance of mental state which may exist, and by its probable effect upon the patient's capacity to undertake the various responsibilities above described. What is required is a lucid commonsense and reasonable appreciation of the situation: no more and no less.

Now that the single ground for *divorce* is establishing to the satisfaction of the judge, that irretrievable breakdown of the marriage has taken place, medical opinions are rarely required in the divorce courts.

Criminal Responsibility

In law, responsibility means liability to punishment. A plea of unsoundness of mind may be raised by way of defence to any criminal charge, but for all practical purposes such a plea is usually confined to charges of murder (this is because for lesser crimes a psychiatric form of disposal may not be advantageous when it may itself lead to long periods of loss of liberty if a Hospital Order is imposed – see below). The law as to responsibility of insane persons is still based upon the answers of the judges consulted by the House of Lords in 1843 after the murder of Mr. Edward Drummond, Private Secretary to Sir Robert Peel. Drummond was shot dead by a man called McNaghten, who was suffering from delusions of persecution. He was tried, and after evidence of his delusions had been heard, was acquitted on grounds of insanity on the judge's direction. The public reaction to this acquittal was most unfavourable and eventually led to a debate in the House of Lords, where a number of questions was put to judges of the High Court. The answers have come to be known as the McNaghten rules, and are in essence as follows:

In order to establish a defence on the grounds of insanity, it must be clearly proved *'that at the time of committing the act the party accused was labouring under such a defect of reason, from disease of the mind, as not to know the nature and quality of the act he was doing, or if he did know it, that he did not know he was doing wrong'*. (Wrong here means contrary to the law.) The second important provision is that if the accused commits an act by reason of delusion, the degree of responsibility which must be attached to him, and therefore in law the degree of culpability which must be attributed, is based upon the justification which the delusion would provide, if it were true. The frank absurdity of evaluating insane delusions as if they were true, while ignoring the underlying mental illness of which the delusions are themselves evidence, has been recognized for over a hundred years; but this aspect of the rules is now rarely invoked.

The principal medical criticisms levelled against the rules are founded upon two points: the first that the rules made no provision for the effect upon conduct of pathological disturbances of emotion, as opposed to disturbance of reason or knowledge; the second that the diagnosis of any kind of insanity is a complex task and cannot be finally entrusted to a panel of laymen, the jury.

In support of the first objection, there is the glaring inadequacy of the rules to take account of the nature of depression, one of the commonest forms of serious mental illness. A depressed patient may be driven by his illness to attempt to commit suicide; but if he has a dependent relative, for example an aged mother, he may kill her first in his mood of utter despair and subsequently be apprehended before he can take his own life. In such a case it is clearly difficult for the honest expert medical witness to maintain either that the man did not know what he was doing, or that he did not know that it was wrong. But the balance of the patient's mind is no less overthrown, and his sanity therefore no less impaired, because the disturbance is primarily emotional rather than rational. The same considerations may apply to a schizophrenic who attacks an innocent person in the delusional belief that he is poisoning him, or to a morbidly jealous man who wounds his spouse in connection with delusions of her infidelity.

However, not all medical objections to the McNaghten rules are themselves free from confusion. Doctors have to remember that the law does not presume to define insanity. That is accepted as a medical question. What the law considers are the conditions which have to be satisfied in order that a person may be excused from criminal responsibility. Moreover the determination of such responsibility, like that of every other question of fact or opinion in the course of trial by jury, must finally be made by the jury themselves. The object of the McNaghten rules is to provide a clear, concise direction for the guidance of judges in advising juries as to the law with regard to criminal responsibility in particular circumstances.

In 1957 the Homicide Act introduced the concept of diminished responsibility, long known in Scotland but almost new to English law, as a potentially mitigating factor, capable of reducing a charge of murder to one of manslaughter. This makes it possible to by-pass the McNaghten rules completely in cases of murder, and diminished responsibility has since that time become by far the commonest psychiatric defence in mitigation in trials for this crime.

The Infanticide Act (1938) had already provided a special offence based on the concept of diminished responsibility, when a mother killed her own infant while the 'balance of her mind' was disturbed in the year after childbirth.

The law on responsibility for an offence committed by a person who is intoxicated by alcohol is in an unsatisfactory state: clearly he might logically defend himself by saying that he was so drunk that he lacked the intent necessary for the alleged offence; but equally clearly if this defence could succeed, drunkards could go scot-free after committing serious crimes, which could not be in accord with public justice.

The Butler report of 1975 proposed that the mandatory life sentence for murder be abolished and maintained that the doctrine of diminished responsibility would then become unnecessary. They proposed a new special verdict 'not guilty on evidence of mental disorder', based on either a) the defendant did not know what he was doing, or b) specific exemption from conviction for defendants suffering from severe mental illness or severe subnormality; and a new offence to deal with people who become violent when voluntarily intoxicated.

Differences of outlook between medicine and the law do not alter the fact that whatever their opinions of the validity of legal concepts as they now exist, medical men, like all other citizens, are bound to respect the law, and to address themselves to comply with it when, for example, they have to give evidence in a particular case.

Doctors called as witnesses must not argue about legal principles, but must confine themselves to elucidation of the facts of the case for the guidance of the court. Any interpretation of the law rests with Her Majesty's judges themselves and nobody else. It is no function of the psychiatrist to argue in court against the law as it stands, however strongly he may feel about it, and in no circumstances should he allow his emotions to colour his judgment on the particular case on which he is engaged.

In the light of the third of the four principles set out at the beginning of this chapter, it is clear that medical evidence about the state of mind of an accused may be in fact of vital importance, and provided that it is given with integrity and objectivity, it will receive the respect and attention of the court.

The Mental Health Act and Individual Liberty

The Mental Health Act of 1959 codifies and supersedes all earlier statutes on the subject, giving this country the benefit of revised and up-to-date law based on the needs of modern psychiatric practice in a humane society. Certain *principles* run throughout the act and embody its spirit. Patients are to be able to seek treatment with no more formality than that required for any other type of illness, so far as possible, so that informal admissions are encouraged as the usual procedure, the courts are not involved (unless there are already criminal proceedings) and all types of hospitals are to be available for psychiatric patients. Those patients who are incapable of appreciating their own need for in-patient treatment in hospital, and who cannot be persuaded to be admitted informally, can be compulsorily admitted for observation or treatment, but only if it is necessary in the interests of their own or other people's health or safety. When this procedure has to be invoked, admission is first recommended by doctors, but a further decision on whether to act on the medical recommendations must be taken by a layman acting on behalf of the patient's over-all interests – either his next-of-kin or a mental welfare officer (a social worker provided by the local authority with an official warrant to act in this capacity).

The success of the intention to encourage informal admission is shown by the fact that on admission to psychiatric units 86 per cent of the patients are of informal status, i.e. free citizens. Many of the other 14 per cent stay on in hospital freely after their short-lasting legal detention expires, so that a survey of the hospitals on any day reveals 94 per cent of the patients being free to leave without formalities.

DEFINITIONS

In England, the whole field of psychiatry is termed 'mental disorder', and is divided into mental illness, subnormality, severe subnormality, psychopathic disorder, and a miscellaneous 'other' category. The legal definitions of the subnormality terms are given in Chapter 15 and of psychopathic personality in Chapter 11. Mental illness is not provided with a statutory definition, so that its meaning will be that in expert professional use at the time.

COMPULSORY ADMISSION FOR OBSERVATION

Section 25 of the Act contains the main provision of Parliament for securing admission for observation in a psychiatric emergency when it is essential. Two medical recommendations are needed, one from a psychiatrist (approved as experienced for this purpose by a Health Authority), and one from any other registered medical practitioner, preferably one with previous experience of the patient (which is to say, that it is desirable but not essential to find the family practitioner if possible). Only one can be on the staff of the admitting hospital; they must examine the patient within 7 days of each other. An application for admission is then needed, by a social worker or the nearest relative, but usually the former is needed in any case, to explain the distressing and disturbing situation to the latter. When the three documents are completed, the patient can be admitted for a period of 28 days for observation. During the twenty-eight days, the patient and the relative cannot insist upon his discharge, but the responsible doctor in the hospital can, and often does, discharge him home if this is indicated on clinical grounds, or can cancel the order, so that the patient remains informally.

The minimum procedure, for use only in emergency, when the two medical recommendations cannot be obtained rapidly, is prescribed under Section 29, when a recommendation by any one doctor and an application by a social worker or any relative, can secure admission for 72 hours, until the fuller procedure can be invoked.

COMPULSORY ADMISSION FOR TREATMENT

This order, under Section 26, also requires two medical recommendations, by a psychiatrist and any other doctor plus an application by the nearest relative, who can refuse to allow the procedure if he chooses to. This order, forcing admission for treatment for up to a year, is a more serious interference with the civil rights of the patient, and accordingly carries additional safeguards. The medical recommendations have to be filled in with more detail of the evidence for the diagnosis and for the statement that admission is 'warranted' (required). The order can be applied to cases of mental illness and severe subnormality at any age, but to subnormality and psychopathic disorder only if the patient is under twenty-one years of age (safeguards because these conditions are hard to define, and shade off into the normal; but compellable when young because the patients then have their greatest chance of benefiting from special treatment or training).

The patients on Treatment orders can be discharged early by their nearest relative, by the responsible medical officer, by the administering Health Authority of the hospital, and by a Mental Health Review Tribunal, to which the patient has a right of direct appeal.

POLICE ORDERS, SECTION 136

Under this section of the Act, a policeman who finds in a public place a person who appears to him to be in need of care or control, can remove him to a place of safety (in practice, a police station or hospital), where he can be detained for up to 72 hours, so that he can be examined by a doctor and interviewed by a social worker, and further arrangements made if necessary. This is a very important provision, as it is the only section of the Act under which a person may lawfully lose his liberty, for alleged mental disorder, without seeing a doctor. It is used 1500 times a year in England; most of the people involved are mentally very disturbed and are correctly and humanely taken to hospital.

DISCHARGE AGAINST MEDICAL ADVICE

Sometimes an informal patient becomes seriously disturbed, and insists on attempting to discharge himself in circumstances in which it would be unsafe, and therefore irresponsible, to allow him to leave hospital precipitately. In these circumstances, an emergency order can be made under Section 29, as described above, or the special procedure for the emergency detention of inpatients, described in Section 30(2) can be invoked. This requires only one form, from the doctor to the hospital administration, and provides authority to keep the patient for up to three days.

Psychiatric Forms of Disposal for Mentally Abnormal Offenders

POLICE DISCRETION

When a person is apprehended while committing a relatively minor offence, and he is obviously mentally unwell, there is a wide degree of informal discretion which can be exercised by the police. For example, a bewildered and hallucinated schizophrenic who steals milk bottles from a doorstep because he is hungry, may simply have arrangements made for him to be readmitted to the local psychiatric unit from which he was discharged before he relapsed. Section 136 of the Mental Health Act, described above, is also used to take abnormal minor offenders to the hospitals which they need.

AT THE BEGINNING OF THE TRIAL

A severely mentally ill patient who cannot understand the proceedings or make a proper defence, may be found 'unfit to plead'. Amnesia does not in itself raise an issue of fitness to stand trial. The trial proceeds no further and the patient is sent to a hospital by order of the Home Secretary.

DURING THE TRIAL

The special verdict of 'not guilty by reason of insanity' in murder trials, the concept of diminished responsibility, and the special cases of infanticide and drunkenness have been discussed above. They are rare issues.

The common provisions for mentally abnormal offenders are Hospital Orders and Probation Orders.

HOSPITAL ORDERS

These can be made at the end of the trial, if the judge or magistrate receives two medical reports, one from an approved psychiatrist, giving a psychiatric diagnosis under the Mental Health Act, and if an order for admission to hospital seems, in all the circumstances, the best way of disposing of the case. The order, under Section 60, is analogous to a Treatment Order – medical disposal is initiated by the two doctors, acted upon by another, non-medical authority, in this case the judge, with the effect that the patient must be in hospital for up to one year, with decisions on treatment being in the hands of the doctor at the hospital.

RESTRICTION ORDER

In about one-fifth of these cases, the judge further makes a Restriction Order under Section 65 of the Act, usually without limit of time, which makes the patient subject to the control of the Home Secretary, in questions of home leave, discharge, and supervision after leaving hospital. This provision protects the public from early discharge of troublesome and dangerous patients.

SPECIAL HOSPITALS

The Special Hospitals (Broadmoor, Rampton, Moss Side and Park Lane in England; Carstairs in Scotland), administered directly by the D.H.S.S. and Scottish Home and Health Department, provide psychiatric treatment in conditions of special security for patients with dangerous, violent or criminal propensities. All of their patients are legally detained, under Treatment Orders or Hospital Orders as just described, or transferred from prison while serving a sentence. The three hospitals in England had in 1975, 2,150 patients.

PSYCHIATRIC PROBATION ORDERS

These may be imposed, with a condition of inpatient or outpatient treatment for a period. The order is a recognition by the court that the offender needs treatment, and gives him the opportunity of receiving it. Although not all patients respond well to treatment under sanctions, the arrangements often work well, especially if doctor and probation officer cooperate fully in their efforts to treat and rehabilitate the patient. The probation order is suitable for exerting some pressure for treatment on some patients with persistent problems which lead to frequently repeated offences, with the eventual prospect of long prison sentences which will be punitive and not reformative. Such patients include the men who repeatedly expose themselves sexually to children or the opposite sex, and alcoholics with repeated offences of drunkenness and vagrancy.

CLINICAL CONDITIONS FOUND AMONG THE
MENTALLY DISORDERED OFFENDERS

These include practically the whole spectrum of psychiatry, although some conditions are more characteristically associated with one type of offence than others. The commonest offences committed by the mentally ill, as by other people, are thefts. Crimes of violence are sometimes committed by schizophrenics in response to delusions, and severely depressed patients may be involved in murders actuated by despairing and merciful motives before the patient's own planned suicide; but many more violent acts are committed by psychopathic personalities with unstable aggressive traits. Sexual offences including indecent exposure, molesting, and attacks on children or adults, are a problem in the management of some mentally handicapped patients, for whom there tends to be an increase in infringements of the law in early adult life, when a somewhat late attainment of sexual maturity may coincide with being too strong physically to be controlled by parents, or with the death of parents who have up until then precariously kept their offspring out of trouble. Arson occasionally is a repetitive problem when committed by the mentally handicapped, although it is also found in many other circumstances. People dependent on drugs are frequently in the courts on charges of illegal possession of drugs and forging prescriptions. Chronic alcoholics sometimes have hundreds of convictions in their record, for drunkenness, fighting, stealing and vagrancy.

Shoplifting is sometimes followed by referral for psychiatric advice when the offender is not a professional thief and appears to have acted in a way that is surprisingly out of character. It is rare for the state of mind to have been such that the accused did not know what she was doing or that it was wrong, but pre-existing states of severe distress or sometimes depressive illness may be found which, while not being capable of securing acquittal, are sometimes very relevant for the attention of the court, so that it can weigh them in the balance when deciding on possibly merciful action, or a measure which ensures that the offender reaches psychiatric care.

Management of Property

The Court of Protection, a branch of the High Court, exists to protect the property and interests of all people who are mentally incapable of managing their own affairs. An application to the Court supported by an appropriate medical recommendation on the form of affidavit obtainable therefrom, is required in any case where the patient, whether in hospital or not, is mentally incapable; this includes the possibility of applying when the patient is only temporarily affected, as by physical illness. The usual procedure is to appoint a receiver to act in the name of and on behalf of the patient, and under the overall supervision of the Court; such a receiver is commonly a close relative, but can be an officer of a local authority. The Court keeps itself informed of the condition of the patient, so that although the arrangements are not subject to time-limit, they can always be terminated on recovery being attested by a medical opinion.

Problems of Consent to Medical Treatment

When emergencies arise with informal patients, there are normally no anxieties about the legal situation, and the staff are indeed justified in feeling that they are correct in, for example, restraining a wildly violent psychiatric patient, for they will be covered by the common law doctrine of necessity.

The legal situation under the Mental Health Act has not been tested in the courts, but the intention of Parliament is clear that the Treatment order under Section 26 is to secure treatment for the patient who requires it. In practice there is great reluctance to proceed beyond nursing care and essential intervention to prevent danger or deterioration, unless there is written informed consent from the patient (provided that he is capable of understanding), or his nearest relative.

Significant Differences in the Law in Scotland

CRIMINAL RESPONSIBILITY

The accused, in a major crime, is examined by two or more independent psychiatrists of national standing on behalf of the Crown, and their findings as to his sanity and fitness to plead are usually accepted by the Crown. Perhaps because of this practice, unfitness to plead appears to be used more frequently in Scotland, and the question of insanity at the time of the crime is raised more rarely. The McNaghten Rules are rarely invoked in Scottish Courts (being essentially an English ruling), but their spirit pervades Scottish judgments as it does those of all English-speaking countries.

DIMINISHED RESPONSIBILITY

This section (Section 2) of the Homicide Act does not apply in Scotland because it has been part of the accepted common law of Scotland for very many years, and in spite of its apparent illogicality, it has worked well. The definition in the Homicide Act is much wider than is accepted in Scottish practice and it has been interesting to note that whereas in England under the new Act many essentially psychopathic individuals have been dealt with under this section, it is rare for a psychopath to be accepted as having diminished responsibility in Scotland.

INDIVIDUAL LIBERTY

It is true to say that both the Mental Health Act 1959 and the Mental Health Scotland Act 1960 are based on the same principles, but there are certain differences between the two Acts. The major differences concern the retention under the Scottish Act of

a) the legal authority for detention, and
b) the central authority.

Authority for the detention of a patient must still have the approval of the Sheriff who may, if he thinks necessary, see the patient and the petitioner and the doctors, and the patient has the right of appeal to the Sheriff against his detention. This has the effect of introducing legal sanction before the patient is committed rather than after he is committed. There is no Mental Health Review Tribunal in Scotland.

The Central Authority is the old Board of Control under another guise and with more limited powers. It is called the Mental Welfare Commission, and consists of seven to nine Commissioners, two of whom must be doctors and one of whom must be a woman.

Its major function is to 'exercise general protective functions on behalf of patients'. This means that the Commissioners are empowered to visit all patients subject to detention, and be available for private interviews if asked by any patient. They also function as an appeal body. They have no power, as the old Board of Control had, to inspect buildings or inspect documents, but require to be informed of the movement of patients subject to detention. They have power to discharge patients and in fact, like the Responsible Medical Officer in Scotland, are required to discharge patients if they think either that they are no longer suffering from mental disorder, or even if they are still suffering from mental disorder, if they can be discharged without danger to their own health and safety or the health and safety of others.

There are very many other minor differences, but the chief one is that of nomenclature. There is no definition of categories in the Scottish Act which says simply 'Mental Disorder in this Act means mental illness or mental defect however caused or manifested'. This in effect leaves these terms to be defined as they are generally understood at whatever time the Act is being operated. By means of a circumlocution within the body of the Act, Scottish legislators have managed to cater for the psychopath and the high-grade defective in exactly the same way as does the English Act without ever mentioning the word psychopath which is perhaps rather clever of them.

Partly because of the scattered rural areas in Scotland and difficulties in communication, the emergency admission is valid for seven days instead of three days. Since the Act came into force this had the effect that many of the patients who are admitted under emergency procedure accept their position in hospital very quickly and no further formal steps need to be taken for their detention. They become quite ready to remain on an informal basis. There is no formal category of admission for observation in Scotland, but because the Responsible Medical Officer must give a report on each patient within twenty-eight days of his admission to justify his further detention, these provisions have the same effect as in the English Act.

MANAGEMENT OF PROPERTY

There is no Court of Protection for patients in Scotland. The Boards of Management are empowered to accept and administer sums of up to £100 on behalf of the patients. Sums over that figure are normally dealt with by the appointment, by the Court of Session, of a Curator Bonis on much the same lines as a Receiver is appointed in England.

References and Further Reading

The Mental Health Act, 1959, 2nd edn, by S. R. Speller, 1964, Institute of Hospital Administrators, is a full and clear guide. The major scholarly work is *Crime and insanity in England*, Volume 1 by Nigel Walker, 1968, and Volume 2 by Nigel Walker and Sarah McCabe 1973, Edinburgh University Press, while for up-to-date discussion and recommendations the *Report of the committee on mentally abnormal offenders*, Chairman Lord Butler, Cmnd. 6244, H.M.S.O. 1975 is indispensable.

A comprehensive survey of the subject-matter of this chapter, at greater length, is 'Psychiatry and the law', by D. Stafford-Clark, in Volume 1 (pp. 431–510) of *Taylor's medical jurisprudence*, 12th edn, Keith Simpson (ed.), 1965, London: Churchill.

Chapter 19

Psychotherapy

Communication and Transformation

For as long as mental illness has been recognized, treatment has been divisible into two main broad headings: they can be called respectively, treatment by attempts at communication, and treatment by attempts at transformation.

Treatment by communication covers all forms of exchange of ideas, discussion, reasoning and emotion: of the effort to reach out into the mind and world of a sick person and, by comprehending it, to make it comprehensible to him: even to enable him to see it in a different way, and to modify his behaviour along lines governed by a deeper and wider understanding and by an increased confidence. This is really the basis of psychotherapy. The term 'psychotherapy' means literally the treatment of the mind. It could therefore logically be applied to all methods of treatment for mental illness. Its use in practice is restricted to those methods which rely for their effect upon the exchange of ideas and understanding between patient and doctor, directed towards relief of the patient's symptoms and distress.

Behaviour therapy, or behaviour modification, was originally born of learning theory, and involved the subtle and painstaking use of training methods to change symptoms which were manifest in the patient's behaviour. Some techniques smacked of transformation of a patient (for example aversion therapy, although even this requires the patient's active and willing consent to enter treatment), but increasingly the emphasis has come to be on long consultations, efforts to understand the patient's world, including his mental world, group and family therapy, and the use of rewards chosen by the patient. It is generally agreed that these forms of treatment now resemble psychotherapy more and more closely.

The field can thus justly be called, as it has been by some of its most active promoters, behavioural psychotherapy. *Treatment by transformation* has a history as long as any form of medical treatment. Its underlying aim is to change the patient by some means which either does not depend at all, or depends only in the most concrete and limited sense, upon the patient's own cooperation, understanding and interest. Under this heading come all the various forms of physical treatment which have been employed to relieve or cure mental illness. The doctor prescribes the treatment because he thinks he knows what will make the patient better, by changing him. The patient need not take part in the treatment but can remain passive, and even relatively detached and uninvolved.

A review of the history of physical treatment in psychiatry shows that an apparently consistent principle of the past has been to inflict some form of unpleasantness or suffering, often in the form of a 'shock' upon the patient as an essential part of treatment, almost as though the patient had to be made to expiate the crime of being mentally ill. Even today this shadow lingers about our attitude to physical treatment. It is necessary therefore to remember that an important aspect of the doctor's task when discussing these forms of treatment with a patient is to disabuse him of the idea that fear or pain, 'shock' or horror play any part in them whatever.

SUPPORTIVE PSYCHOTHERAPY

Psychotherapy can be of two main kinds, depending upon whether the object of communication between patient and doctor is purely support to sustain the patient, or whether it is to effect some change in his personality or attitude towards his present difficulties, by interpretation of his feelings and predicament which may lead to a better understanding. Supportive psychotherapy and interpretive psychotherapy, which may also be called insight therapy, differ therefore considerably in technique. The former is usually simpler, less ambitious in aim, easier in execution and indicated primarily for patients for whom a more ambitious approach would be impracticable or unproductive.

Nevertheless supportive psychotherapy plays a great part in outpatient management of patients who might otherwise receive no help whatever from their doctor. It can include direct, simple and sympathetic advice, and sheer reassurance and encouragement; and may be combined with practical intervention in the social circumstances of the patient, whereby emotional complications of his family life or employment are constructively modified through personal contact with the family or employer, sometimes in liaison with a social worker.

The foundation for supportive psychotherapy of this kind, which is frequently combined with appropriate medicinal symptomatic treatment, is of course a comprehensive history, on which emphasis has already been laid (see Chapter 2). Following such a history it should be possible for the doctor to gain an understanding of the patient in some ways more objective and comprehensive than that perhaps ever gained by any other single person, including, of course, the patient himself. Such a comprehensive picture of the patient and the general direction and significance of the tendencies revealed in his life should enable the doctor in this early stage to form a sound idea of the genesis of the patient's symptoms, and the ways in which the stresses to which he has been subjected may be lightened or relieved.

Thereafter such advice or explanation as the doctor has to offer will be based not upon his own personal feelings about the desirability of any particular solution; still less upon a projection on his part of what he would do if he were in the patient's shoes: these being the two shortcomings from which so much well-intentioned lay advice so often suffers. By contrast, the doctor's advice and explanation will be based upon his objective assessment of the patient's individual needs and possibilities, gained from his knowledge of the patient acquired in the way described, and accepted without prejudice of any kind.

He may also consider that the patient will require periodic advice and supervision for some time, in order that the readjustment which is desirable may be followed up and consolidated. From the patient's point of view, the knowledge that there exists somebody who not only understands him and his symptoms, but who is able to accept him without hostility and distress, to explain to him the nature of his difficulties and their connection with symptoms which he has developed, and to help and support him through the stresses which underlie these symptoms, is in itself a very great help and comfort. It may enable such a patient to resume work and domestic responsibility which have formerly proved impossible, and to take his place once again as an active member of the community. Treatment of this kind represents the first line of defence against mental illness which the medical profession has to offer; and much of the avoidable unhappiness caused by fear, anxiety, tension or guilt in daily life, is often successfully relieved or prevented in this way. Supportive psychotherapy can be conducted on the basis of interviews of up to half an hour once a week, a fortnight, or every three or four weeks. Often it is quite unnecessary to acquaint the patient with more than a fraction of the underlying implications which the detailed study of his life has revealed; but as a basis for any kind of advice, explanation or reassurance, insight on the part of the doctor, as accurate and complete as his skill and training can render it, is indispensable.

Psychotherapy of this limited but invaluable kind should be within the capacity of every practising doctor. The expenditure of a limited amount of time in this way is not only humane, but economical; for by the skilled use of a few hours spread out over weeks or months, the physician may not only avert the chronic invalidism and demoralization of the neurotic patient, but may also spare himself the bitterness and frustration which inevitably assail a practitioner continually confronted with this aspect of human suffering, who has never acquired the interest or understanding necessary to deal with it effectively.

INTERPRETIVE PSYCHOTHERAPY

All interpretive psychotherapy is based on three principles. They are:

1 Behaviour is prompted chiefly by emotional considerations, but insight and understanding are necessary to modify and control such behaviour, and the aims underlying it.

2 A very significant proportion of human emotion, together with the action to which it leads, is not normally accessible to personal introspection, being rooted in areas of the mind which are beneath the surface of consciousness.

3 It follows logically (and is supported empirically by experimental and clinical work) that *any process which makes available to individual consciousness the true signficance of emotional conflicts and tensions hitherto repressed*, will thereby produce both heightened awareness, and increased stability and emotional control.

The application of these principles in practice can lead not simply to improved health in its widest sense, but also to a more mature and developed personality.

Nevertheless, psychotherapy aimed at providing insight into his own conscious and unconscious life, and into the deeper relationship of symptoms to emotional conflict, is clearly a less comfortable and acceptable sort of treatment for the patient himself, at any rate in the early stages. Yet it offers the considerable advantage of enabling him to achieve an awareness of himself which will not only help to arm him against present difficulties, but will make it easier for him to control at least a part of his fate in the future. It is less comfortable because the patient has to accept from the outset a larger share of the responsibility for the success of the treatment, and to experience to a greater degree the painful effect of examining his own emotionally tender spots. It is also a more difficult form of treatment for the doctor since it imposes a considerable strain upon him as well as the patient, and does not permit him to relieve his anxiety about the patient by taking the patient's fears out of his own control.

The original, classical, and most elaborate form of this treatment was that developed by Freud, and called by him psychoanalysis. Analytical psychotherapy, developed by Jung, and individual psychotherapy, by Adler, are two further specialized psychotherapeutic techniques, worked out by former pupils of Freud who later diverged from him to create their own approach to the goal of self-awareness. They will be briefly described.

The advantage claimed exclusively for methods of analytic treatment by their proponents is that when completed they are radical and exhaustive. What has been spent in time has been repaid in depth and degree of awareness and consequent stability. In practice a full analysis demands not less than three to five interviews a week for anything from two to four years, excluding only the inevitable breaks caused by holidays and absence of doctor or patient. Any procedure which demands so much expenditure of skilled time is inevitably costly. Moreover such procedures are suitable only for patients whose intelligence, determination, and resources of time or money, are sufficient to enable them to complete and profit from so intensive a course of treatment.

They are thus highly selective and self-limiting forms of treatment and moreover can be practised safely and successfully only by those whose training has fulfilled certain rigorous conditions. But despite these limitations, they are procedures of great importance. This importance derives not simply from results gained in individually suitable patients, but from the body of knowledge which these methods have contributed to psychopathology, and most of all from the application of both the knowledge and the methods in modified form to the evolution of various techniques of briefer psychotherapy devoted to the attainment of insight, but aimed at providing this, at least in its immediate essentials, within a matter of weeks or months, by means less expensive in time and money.

The historical development of the psychotherapies will be traced briefly later in this chapter, with a fuller account of brief psychotherapy.

PSYCHO-ANALYSIS

The initial interviews follow the same general pattern as those of any other psychotherapeutic procedure. So far as possible the history must be obtained and noted in an orderly and comprehensible way in the analyst's records. Thereafter it is the task of the patient to produce, out loud and absolutely without suppression or selection of any kind, all his thoughts and feelings about whatever is uppermost in his mind. This is the method called 'free association'. It may sound difficult, but in practice it is even more difficult than it sounds, at least in the early stages of treatment.

Offered the hitherto inconceivable opportunity of acknowledgment and expression, many of the ideas which rise into the patient's mind are thrust down almost before he has had time to become aware of them; and this of course is preconscious rather than truly conscious material. How much more difficult still is that acknowledgment of the underlying source of such ideas, which can only be achieved with time, practice, and above all, a confidence which at the outset no patient can possibly have.

The nature of the immediate practical difficulties of conforming to this one essential rule of procedure, namely that nothing shall be suppressed and nothing selected, demands that every possible measure which helps the patient to do his part of the work be adopted. It is for this reason that patients are encouraged to lie down, to relax completely, to look at nothing more exciting than the ceiling, and to talk without the visible presence of another person to distract them. The analyst sits out of their range of vision, and while they are able to continue their part of the job, may have no cause for intervention of any kind. But all the time the analyst is recording, sorting, and studying the material produced, bearing in mind its possible interpretations and its correlation with what has gone before, so that as the analysis proceeds he accumulates a deeper source of understanding the patient which he does not obtrude into the process, but uses only when, without help, the patient cannot go further.

Inevitably and repeatedly any patient conscientiously doing his best in this way encounters resistance in his own mind, violent feelings which he cannot or dare not pursue further, and often finds, when approaching the outer defences of some long-buried painful memory or feeling, that he cannot go on. We know from our brief survey of normal psychology and psychopathology that much of what must inevitably cause him difficulty and distress will date from the earlier personal relationships which have been connected with intense and conflicting emotion. The release of such emotion in the course of treatment, before its source has reached awareness or been understood and accepted, is in itself intensely disturbing, and the patient instinctively and unconsciously seeks to rationalize or project the emotion which he feels. Under the conditions of treatment the person who is inevitably selected for the rationalization or projection is the analyst.

In this way during the course of treatment the patient comes to feel the love and hatred, the dependence and the rebellion, rivalry or rejection towards the analyst, that he has felt but never fully acknowledged for other people in his life; people whose impact has been earlier and inescapably close; people such as his parents, his first love, or his friends and enemies, heroes and villains of his childhood. This uncritical and barely understood investment of emotion in the person conducting the treatment is called the transference. The control of this transference, regulation of its depth and intensity, are to a great extent in the hand of the analyst, since he has the underlying interpretation available for use as the occasion demands. To interpret or interfere with the transference too early is to deprive it of the strength necessary to enable the patient to carry on with his already difficult contribution to the treatment. It is also, at a deeper level, to imply a tendency on the part of the analyst to escape from the obligation of his part in treatment, and may even spring from his own anxiety or insecurity if this has not been adequately dealt with in the course of his training. But to interpret inadequately or too late, or to fail to deal with the transference situation at all, is to risk the development of a total dependence on the part of the patient which may be a more serious complication than the illness with which he presented himself.

The handling of the transference situation is thus of vital importance in the course of psycho-analysis, as indeed in the course of all forms of psychotherapy. It is the existence of the transference which both enables the patient to discover the nature of his underlying feelings and then to acknowledge them. Once this has been done he often finds himself able to regard them in a far more tolerant and dispassionate light, and so be liberated not simply from their effect upon his past but from their influence upon his future.

JUNGIAN ANALYSIS: ANALYTICAL PSYCHOLOGY

The technique of analytical psychology as originated by Jung differs from the original technique of psycho-analysis in that far less emphasis is placed upon free association, and much more importance attached to an analysis and interpretation of certain aspects of the patient's fantasies and dreams, which are handled in a way quite different from that propounded by Freud, in his approach to the analysis of dreams by association. Perhaps the essential difference between Jung's and Freud's concept of unconscious mental life is that while the Freudian view maintains that the unconcious mind contains essentially only instinctual drives and repressed complexes, the Jungian thesis is that there is an enormous reservoir of shared unconscious wisdom and experience throughout the whole of humanity, which permeates each individual unconscious mind, and may enter consciousness only in symbolic form to influence thought and behaviour in powerful but indirect ways. The symbolic forms taken by these powerful archaic mental processes, regarded as common to the entire human race, are called archetypes: and it is in the archetypal nature of myths, art, stories, and dreams, that the Jungian analyst finds the clue to his patient's problems and their interpretation.

The projection of emotion into the relationship between analyst and doctor is analysed, although there is emphasis on the joint struggle by both of them to cure the patient. Jung's religious and philosophical interests meant that he did not shrink from discussing the meaning of life and death with the patient, nor from talking of the healing of the soul.

Some of the difference in interests of the two men can be understood by comparing the titles of the books they wrote on the twentieth-century predicament: Freud wrote of 'Civilization and its discontents', Jung of 'Modern man in search of a soul'.

ADLERIAN ANALYSIS: INDIVIDUAL PSYCHOLOGY

Adler's special contribution to individual psychotherapy was to stress the importance of the drive towards power, which lies at the heart of so much human endeavour.

He observed that for many people the achievement of power, status and prestige, was at least as important as the search for sexual gratification, and could produce as significant an impact upon the individual's life and emotional development. It was Adler who was responsible for the immortal phrase 'inferiority complex'; meaning not a conscious feeling of inferiority, but rather an unconscious constellation of ideas characterized by an intolerable sense of insecurity and inadequacy, of which the subject is largely unaware. The effect of such a complex upon behaviour is by contrast to produce a somewhat assertive attitude and to drive the individual into situations wherein he must prove his deeper misgivings to be false.

Adlerian analysis concentrates attention upon the patient's idealized, partly conscious, concept of himself, and the goals which he has set himself; and seeks to relate these to his actual personality, and to the existent circumstances, opportunities, and limitations of his life. In the inevitable conflicts and frustrations implicit in the gulf between aspiration and achievement, are the foundations either of pathological emotion and behaviour, or of renewed and constructive endeavour. By interpretation and insight, Adlerian analysis aims at enabling the individual to become aware of the true springs of his own needs, drives, and impulses, and where these are compensatory to some real or imagined weakness in himself, to evaluate their implications consciously and by discriminating between valid and invalid goals, free himself to pursue the one and discard the other.

The content of an Adlerian analysis is therefore essentially related more to the relationship of the patient's personal aspirations and goals of achievement, both conscious and unconscious, and to his social setting and total life situation, than the more instinctual sexual fulfilment which Freud saw as the ultimate driving force in human experience, or the integration of the personality, which remains Jung's concept of human fulfilment.

Obviously an account as concise as this, summarizing essentially the outlines of the analytical techniques, cannot go into the details of the psychodynamic theories underlying them. But enough has been said to indicate the highly complicated nature of this kind of treatment, and therefore the inaccuracy of using the terms 'psycho-analysis' or even 'analysis' for psychiatric interviews which may have as their goal nothing more fundamental than the clarification of some immediate personal problem or domestic situation. In fact the vast majority of psychiatric interviews are of this relatively limited nature; and treatment by psycho-analysis, Jungian analysis or Adlerian analysis is suitable for only a very small proportion of patients who require psychotherapy in some form or another.

Historical Development of the Psychotherapies

While the student and doctor do not require a detailed knowledge of the different forms of psychotherapy in use today, a brief account tracing the development of the main forms may be helpful, even though it cannot do justice to the recent great increase in enterprise in this field.

The ancestor of all the psychotherapies was of course Freud's invention of psychoanalysis, a towering, highly original achievement. Freud's theories changed considerably during his long life, and not all his different theories can be reconciled with each other. A tradition of orthodox psychoanalysis firmly in the line of descent from Freud's work persists to this day, with training and practice in many countries. There have been developments even within the orthodox school, however.

The emphasis has tended to shift from concern with the effects of unconscious instinctual life to '*ego-psychology*', in which the spotlight is more on how the conscious portion of the personality is organized in coping, through defences, with the demands of conscience, unconscious material and the external world. Freud's youngest daughter Anna Freud wrote the influential book '*The ego and the mechanisms of defence*' (1937) on this subject, and she also developed the application of psychoanalysis to young children. She believed, too, that the parent's attitude to the child was as important as the other forces. There have been further developments of theory, especially by Fairbairn and Winnicott. Melanie Klein developed a distinct body of theory and practice, which remains a minority faction of psychoanalysis. She claimed to analyse, using play, even younger children, under the age of six, and emphasized the importance of innate aggressive drives in early infancy in the formation of the child's personality.

In America, social and cultural influences tended to be allowed for and were woven into the theories of the widely read Karen Horney (e.g. *'Self-analysis'*, *'The neurotic personality of our time'*, and papers expounding the social rather than the biological influences on female personality), and Erich Fromm (e.g. *'The fear of freedom'* and many discussions of sociology and politics). Psychoanalysis and its developments, including the breakaway Adlerian group which scarcely developed further, remained very dominant in American psychiatry until well into the 1960s.

Jungian analytical psychotherapy has been discussed above – since its original development it has remained a vigorous discipline, with professional bodies for training and psychotherapy.

Another heretical early psychoanalyst was Wilhelm Reich, who became interested in the psychological effects of political repression, and in the nature of the orgasm. His therapy was directed to relieving inhibitions which he believed became fixed in the character and in the bodily posture of the patient. Achievement of a perfect orgasm became all-important as a sign of health. Reich became psychotic himself, and would have been almost forgotten but for a recent revival of interest in the body in psychotherapy (mentioned below).

The pure gold of psychoanalysis, however, had to be alloyed with base metal from early in its history, and great efforts have gone into developing shorter forms of psychotherapy using some of the same body of theory, and hoping to achieve worth-while results in attaining limited goals. For example, one influential psychotherapist has been Carl Rogers, who calls his practice *client-centred therapy*. He sets few conditions, peddles very little theory, and emphasizes the attitude of the therapist. He says that if the therapist accurately perceives the patient's thoughts and behaviour, if he has empathy for the patient's feelings and regards him with 'unconditional positive regard', then the stage is set for helping him, regardless of exact orientation or technique. Our own account of brief psychotherapy is given after this section.

It must also be remembered that the *'case-work'* taught to the social work profession has been based on the psychodynamic principles of psychoanalysis, applied in simplified form, and is thus also one of the descendants of Freud's work, even though other approaches, and social theory, are increasingly applied at the same time.

Transactional analysis, a new therapy devised by Eric Berne, is a descendant of psychoanalysis, with a very much simplified body of theory, intellectualized, schematic, non-emotional and very clear. The personality is divided into three aspects, personifications of Parental, Adult and Childlike features, which are evidently transformations, albeit not exact, of respectively, Freud's superego, ego, and id, although the Child is a much wider concept, including for example, playfulness. The theory and method have proved to be adaptable and powerful tools, in individual and especially group therapy, and they are easy to teach to pupils and patients. The movement came from America and is taking root here rapidly.

Another source of present psychotherapies has been *behaviour therapy*, developed originally from the application of experimental learning theory to human behaviour. The scientific approach, and the high value put upon the evaluation of results, have remained, as the practice has expanded and has discovered many new applications for itself. The combination of psychotherapy with science, and without medical techniques, was very attractive to the clinical psychologists, who took it up enthusiastically. This emphasis has remained, although teaching the methods to nurses is proving very successful, and more doctors are learning the techniques too, sometimes combining them with drugs or other physical methods.

Group therapy had only tenuous roots before the Second World War, but has become increasingly influential ever since. The development of *therapeutic communities* dates from the work of Maxwell Jones in founding what is now the Henderson Hospital specializing in the community treatment of patients with psychopathic personalities. The concept fertilized the open-door policy in mental hospitals in the 1950s, and led to increasing attention being paid to the social structure of wards and of the hospital as a whole. A further influence has been exerted by sociological writings on institutions, especially '*Asylums*' (1961), which emphasized what Goffman found wrong with mental hospitals. Community meetings of staff and patients in wards, and even open meetings of the whole staffs of hospitals, have become standard practice in many fields, especially in wards and day hospitals treating patients

with neurotic and personality disorders, and in adolescent units.
Therapeutic communities of specialized types, usually emphasizing
vigorously honest confrontations and intense social pressure, have
been common experimental approaches in the rehabilitation of
drug addicts and recidivist criminals with severe personality
disorders.

Small group psychotherapy also traces its influence in this
country back to pioneers in the early postwar period, in the
Northfield Military Hospital. It then passed via the Tavistock clinic
to psychiatry at large. Bodies of theory were worked out by the
pioneers, with greater or less connection with psychoanalysis, social
psychology and systems theory, all of which have influenced the
increasing application of group methods to psychotherapy. Nowadays all psychiatric services, clinical psychologists and trained
social workers spend some of their psychotherapeutic effort in
group work, and simpler forms of counselling and support are
often conducted similarly.

Behaviour therapy, originally like psychoanalysis an individual
technique, is sometimes practised in groups, although the emphasis
is then on treating a collection of individuals together rather than
the group process.

Further contributions have come via social psychology and
drama, in the form of the widespread use of *role-playing* in individual and group psychotherapy, as well as *psycho-drama*. Psycho-
drama was the invention of one man, J. L. Moreno, but now is
influencing others of the experimental psychotherapies.

A further trend towards concentrating on the patient's and
therapist's present feelings, and on openness, honesty, and lack of
socially-induced inhibition, has led to *Gestalt* therapy, individual
or in groups, employing 'games' and emotional exercises. There
are many unsafe fringe activities calling themselves psychotherapy
and resulting from a brew of: a fashionable preoccupation with
the body and its relaxation; an equally fashionable disinhibition and
lack of restraint; the current cult of irrationalism; and sheer
charlatanry.

Encounter groups originated in staff training and outside clinical
services, and they remain mainly a mode of staff training, and of
course a spare-time activity of people who are not patients. There
is, however, considerable overlap with small group psychotherapy
and Gestalt therapy.

Family therapy, twenty years old in the United States in the hands of dedicated specialists, has become common here in the past few years only. The intellectual prerequisite is the theory that most if not all psychiatric disorders are disorders not *of* people but *between* people, and this is used in various theories with admixtures of traditional psychoanalysis and of systems theory. The founders of family therapy, especially in the U.S.A., have not been group therapists, although it is in one sense a form of group therapy with a small, intense, naturally occurring group. Behaviour modification methods are also frequently used in treating families, and in marital therapy.

Marital therapy, increasingly requested and increasingly prescribed, is also expanding rapidly, concurrently, and using the same methods as in treating families with children. Some of the *sexual therapeutic methods* are described in Chapter 12.

There are threads running through this historical account of the changes in the types of psychotherapy used to help patients. At first the patient's past was the target which was to be reached by way of the technique of psychoanalysis, but increasingly the concern has become with present relationships and immediate thoughts and feelings – the so-called 'here-and-now'. The mode has changed from abstract discussion to present emotion and increasingly is coming to involve the body and relaxation. The relationship between doctor and patient has changed in formality from Freud sitting behind the couch, to doctor facing patient across the consulting-room desk, to doctor and patient in armchairs, to the doctor leading a group; on to sitting on the floor in encounter groups with an informally dressed doctor freely recounting his own problems. The disorder to be tackled was seen at first to be in the patient, then increasingly it was identified as being between people in the family, and the family is often being identified as the emotionally disordered unit. Debate has started, especially in America, about whether society causes the problems in the families, and whether therefore the psychotherapy should not logically be directed to changing society, with psychiatrists cast as social reformers.

BRIEF METHODS OF INTERPRETIVE (OR INSIGHT) THERAPY

All brief methods of insight therapy depend for their brevity upon reduction of two main elements which normally comprise a considerable part of psycho-analytic procedure, and absorb much of the time involved. These two elements are the repetition involved in working through problems against resistance, while relying solely upon the patient's free associations to bring these problems back into the field of exploration every time they are evaded or shelved, and also the time and effort consumed in dealing with comparatively irrelevant material, and in coming to the point in material which is unquestionably important but too emotionally charged to be readily handled by the patient.

The essence of all methods of brief psychotherapy is therefore in some way to select those areas of the patient's life which are most relevant to the problems he faces and the symptoms he displays, and having selected them to focus the entire procedure upon them until they have been dealt with, and the necessary changes thereby effected in the mental life of the patient. Techniques of this kind are on the whole harder to acquire and to practise successfully even than the methods of full-scale analysis; there are a number in existence, but only a few have proved their worth. The need for them, provided that they are consistent and dependable in competent hands, is unquestionable.

Training is needed, so that the therapist has knowledge of his own personality and of his blind spots and prejudices in relationships. Without this knowledge he cannot deploy his personality accurately in his efforts to understand and help the patient.

All these methods have in common the paring down of the analytical procedure to deal exclusively with the immediate or essentially alterable sources of complaint. The criticism sometimes offered by orthodox analysis of such methods is that they tend to patch rather than to recreate the personality of the patient. The answer to this criticism must be that the resources of medicine as a whole are in practice inevitably compelled to do just that and no more, to as many people as possible. Moreover the perfectionist attitude implicit in so dogmatic an approach cannot claim to be supported by the results of full-scale analysis, in any but a minute proportion even of those for whom it is practicable.

In practice a useful framework for brief psychotherapy can be constructed by planning with the patient eight to a dozen interviews at weekly intervals, each of thirty to forty-five minutes duration, for which the following targets are set:

1 Establishment of rapport; effective doctor/patient relationship: adequate history (for two interviews). This can lead to an

appreciation of the situation – using the word appreciation here
in its military sense.

2 Selection of goals; formulation of overall plan of treatments;
exploration of goal (subsequent three to four interviews).

3 Interpretation of material (begun at appropriate stages of
exploratory interviews, but completed within context of overall
treatment); integration of these interpretations with the patient's
own concept of his life situation and its implications; recognition and acceptance by the patient, support and reassurance by
doctor (final three to four interviews).

The methods, mechanisms, and special techniques involved, are
indicated in the table below:

	Methods:		*Mechanisms*	*Special Techniques*
	Patient	*Doctor*		
Ventilation:	Describes symptoms	Listens	Internal & Passive	Abreactive
70%		Accepts	(Stress Reaction	
		Encourages	dissolves)	
Exploration:	Recalls trauma	Questions	Internal & Active	Analytic
20%	Discovers connections	Interprets	(Stress Reaction	
			resolved by patient)	
Guidance:	Listens	Reassurance	External & Passive	Counselling
10%	Comments	Explanation	(Stress or Reaction	Suggestion
	Questions	Advice	reduced by doctor)	Social aid

As a general rule, it is reasonable to regard the relative proportion of these three contributions of ventilation, exploration, and
guidance in the total course of treatment as being respectively,
70 per cent, 20 per cent and 10 per cent. The initial interviews
should consist essentially in the acceptance by the doctor of the
patient's need to communicate, and to be understood. It is not
what the doctor tells the patient but what the doctor permits the
patient to tell him, in the early interviews, which is likely to be
decisive in the success or failure of treatment of this kind.

Selection for individual interpretive psychotherapy has been
very little studied, yet although it is naturally an individual matter,
there is much agreement on the main points. Curiosity by the
patient about how his own personality works, an ability to talk in
and understand abstract terms, and a willingness to proceed with
psychological treatment even when the doctor predicts that it will

be hard work and sometimes painful, are all required. For psychoanalysis, as mentioned above, they need to be present in high degree. Where the doctor, in an assessment interview, detects unwillingness to change or inability to change, for example because of a deadlocked life situation or because of advancing age, he will tend to recommend supportive treatment or other methods. In the first interview, a trial interpretation of behaviour or a pattern of behaviour in terms of emotional conflict will help in assessing the patient's suitability: it will be observed whether the patient understands the medium of interpretation, and takes to it, or whether he is unable to see the point, or is defensive against it.

LARGE GROUPS AND THE THERAPEUTIC COMMUNITY

The principles of the therapeutic community are that communications should be so free and open as to reduce tensions, and that feedback to the members on how they affect each other can be used to help the patients (and perhaps the staff) to change. If the members are together for much of the time, then the community (such as a ward or day hospital) could be a powerful instrument studying and using interpersonal problems. To do this successfully, all the members of the community must attend the meetings and must be ready to participate, even the doctors and leaders. Communications are more free when the staff show that they are willing to forgo their privileged position so far as possible, such as by joining in the meetings and not wearing uniform.

It becomes necessary to study all the events of the community in meetings, to avoid the tense effects of private relationships off-stage: privacy is a casualty of therapeutic communities. Staff meetings are required in which, again, roles are discussed in ways relatively uninhibited by traditional hierarchies. The therapeutic community is the progenitor of the current concept of the 'multi-disciplinary team' in psychiatric units, in which decisions are made rather more democratically than heretofore.

There are many unresolved problems, however. The team cannot be completely democratic when the medical member has inalienable legal responsibility for the care of the patients, and indeed the importance of the role of the leader in therapeutic communities has not yet been fully worked out. Many of the well-known ones have in fact thrived with strong leaders. The democratic intentions and thrust of the approach are clear, but little is known about its results, and there are dangers of anarchy and of neglect of standards of traditional care and of other methods of treatment. These cautions apply less cogently when the setting is not a medical one, as in communities for rehabilitating addicts and criminals. Some of these communities have experimented with meetings of a special kind, developing an expectation of crudely frank confrontations of each other's weakness of personality, only physical violence being barred. The emotional effect of such peer-group pressure in a closed community is very great; it could be, but is not proved to be, beneficial to some people. Research on results is needed, and bearing in mind that these communities are highly selective about whom they take in, it should pay attention to excluded groups, too.

In general psychiatric units, however, the routine of full ward meetings can be used in such a way as to be helpful. Issues of general interest to the ward, and causing tension and disturbed behaviour, can be aired, understood, and perhaps resolved in fruitful ways. For example an unpopular noisy patient is discussed, his problems hinted at or mentioned, the other patients express their resentment at being kept awake, and the result may be different arrangements for the following night, better understanding all round, less tension, and fewer requests for hypnotic drugs. Difficulties over tensions between patients and staff may be resolved in this way, too, staff meetings being needed at the same time to discuss the ward meeting and to be aware of tensions among the staff which may be relevant to the work of the ward.

SMALL GROUP PSYCHOTHERAPY

A number of different theoretical bases have been put forward for use in the understanding of therapeutic groups, and these have varied from regarding the process as akin to psychotherapy of a number of patients who have been brought together but remain individuals, to concentrating exclusively on the processes of the group as a group, in which few or no comments are made on individuals. Although an element of time-saving persists, with group pyschotherapy inevitably being seen as an economical way of giving psychotherapy to a number of patients at once (always provided that they can be substantially helped when seen as a group), most of the present use of group methods depends on the theories and practice that use the group processes themselves as particular ingredients in a prescribed form of psychotherapy.

Factors for selection for group psychotherapy include symptoms mainly in the field of social anxiety, and social effectiveness, as well as problems with maintaining successful relationships. Curiosity, persistence, commitment and some degree of articulateness are needed, as for individual psychotherapy. Unsuitable patients include those who have never had a settled relationship in their lives, people whose social isolation borders on paranoid psychosis, and other very disturbed personalities who, if suitable for psychotherapy at all, need very carefully conducted individual treatment. Psychopathic personalities, too, can be expected to be disruptive in a group, at the same time as not profiting from it.

Approximately eight patients sit in a circle, with a leader and often a co-leader, meeting for an hour and a half weekly. It is possible to plan a fixed period of treatment from the beginning, in which all those who begin are expected to remain (a 'closed' group), or to continue indefinitely with some newcomers and departures from time to time (an 'open' group). The original selection of the patients clearly has a considerable effect on what comes to pass as the group gets to work: it can be arranged for homogeneity (for example: all male indecent exposers), or usually for mixture of sexes, ages and kinds of symptoms. It is important to avoid isolating any patient as the only homosexual, the only unmarried person, the only black, and so forth.

Preliminary rules are punctuality, an obligation to keep confidential what happens in the group, and an obligation not to meet socially outside the group. There is no explicit task given the group, only the implicit one to be a group together in the process of getting better, and to talk in an uncensored way (compare the 'free association' in psychoanalysis).

In these circumstances the talk comes to be increasingly in the form of the patients' responses to each other. An infinitely complicated system of relationships and responses builds up between all the individuals in the room and also concerning the atmosphere and intentions of the group itself as a social entity. There is pressure on the leader to give directions, suggest topics and answer questions, which he resists, as, if he complies, the group will degenerate into social chit-chat.

The leader has responsibility for the safety of the members of the group, who have to be protected from harmful pressure, sexual involvements which will be damaging, and relentless scapegoating.

He does this by interpreting what is happening, supporting the patient who is becoming isolated, monitoring the degree of tension in the group, distinguishing between silences which are fruitful and thoughtful and those that are over-long and threatening, and with similar interventions.

The members of the group participate in a rich interchange of personal reactions which become increasingly spontaneous and candid as social defences are lowered progressively during the life of the group. They may be encouraged by finding other members who share the same secret feelings of shame and inadequacy. They may gain new insights into themselves through the comments on how they appear to the others, and may, with encouragement, try out new forms of behaviour, inconceivable before, within the support of the group. Tasks may be suggested, to be attempted between meetings, with eager interest at the next meeting as to how the experiment came out.

In general, the subject is a many-sided and complex one, and even less than individual psychotherapy can it be taught satisfactorily to students from books. This account is the briefest introduction, and must be supplemented by reading from the list of recommended books given at the end of this chapter, and by indispensable further training, before group psychotherapy can be attempted.

Group counselling stands in approximately the same relationship to group psychotherapy as does brief psychotherapy to interpretive psychotherapy. The members are selected because they need help with a specific problem or group of problems, and the theme of the talk in the group can correctly be allowed to revolve around practical issues and conscious responses between the members. The leader, while being aware of tensions and transference problems, tends not to interpret them but rather to lead away from them.

The *results* of group psychotherapy have not been very clearly evaluated yet. Many patients report having been helped, by a variety of different styles of group treatment, and a substantial number fail to be helped at all: by the very nature of the treatment they frequently drop out of the group fairly early in its history. These patients are apparently not harmed by it, but it is true that their fate is not systematically studied. The patients who remain report a wide variety of factors as having been, in their opinion, conducive to their improvement, especially the feeling of strong support in the group, and the revelation of their own secret thoughts after great struggles.

ENCOUNTER GROUPS AND TRAINING GROUPS

Groups of individuals working in organizations, and including the staff of psychiatric units, have met regularly for the express purpose of training in sensitivity to the emotions of other people, and for increasing skill in understanding others. The leaders encourage sincere, frank and free reactions to each other among the members, and the expectation has now developed that this will happen. As a result, it does happen, actively encouraged by 'games', the study of non-verbal communication, role-playing each other and little dramas enacted in the group. Part of the ambience of the dropping of customary reserve and rituals between people is an encouragement of bodily contact and massage. Present emotion tends to be greatly magnified especially when the groups meet frequently or for long individual sessions, with abreaction of anger and unhappiness. Discussions of, and interest in past history for its own sake, tend to be discouraged, as they damp down the heightening emotions.

The movement now contains a wide variety of styles. Discussion groups of staff, or 'T-groups' (T for training) with responsible skilled leaders, and eschewing emotionalism for its own sake, may well be able to develop the sensitivity and skill of the members when they relate to other people. The formation of encounter groups for 'personal growth', as a spare-time fashion, however, can be a dangerous matter with unselected members or unsuitable leaders.

Most of the participants feel at the end of an intensive series of groups that they have had an enriching and fulfilling experience, which has changed them lastingly for the better. This is usually very transient, however, and follow-up results show that much is a short-lived euphoria, which has gone a few months later. Moreover a tenth of participants are seriously upset, with the possibility of permanent emotional harm. It must be assumed for the moment that, at least with seriously distressed people, encounter groups are likely to be dangerous.

GENERAL PRACTITIONER (BALINT) GROUPS

The holding of seminars of general practitioners, with a psycho-therapist as leader, in order to become better psychotherapists in the course of studying their doctor-patient relationships, originated with Michael Balint, and was described in his book *'The doctor his patient and the illness'*. The movement's popularity has grown has outlived its founder, and seems likely to grow further.

The participants recount their cases and their responses to them. Light comes to be thrown on the influence of the doctor's training in medicine, his traditional interest in physical diagnoses and meticulous care in excluding them by physical investigations, and on the powerful effect on the patient of the doctor's deeply held convictions on illness, suffering and how patients should behave. His feelings about which patients are interesting, which attractive, which deserving, are found to be influencing every consultation. Patients tend to 'offer' complaints of illness, tentatively, and sensitive doctors continue listening to the offers and gently exploring their origins, before allowing the offers to 'organize' into an illness, which can limit the doctor's scope of vision into the patient's life as a whole.

In one vivid phrase after another, Balint illuminates the doctor-patient relationship in general practice, starting his book from a discussion of our relative ignorance of the pharmacology of the drug 'doctor', the most important drug we have, and concluding: ' "Advice" is usually a well-intentioned shot in the dark, is nearly always futile, and that applies even more strongly to "reassurance". We have found that it is more profitable both for doctors and patients to diagnose the problem; more often than not, when that is done there will be no need either for advice or for reassurance. The real problem is likely to be unpleasant or even painful, but it will be real, and with hard work it is probable that something real can be done about it'.

FAMILY THERAPY

The interest in family therapy is not merely a new method of treatment but a sign of a major philosophical shift in how psychiatric disorders are construed by those consulted about them. The traditional care of all good doctors to know about the patient's family in order to understand their effect on the patient, and his effect on them, is now seen to be insufficient. The patient's illness may be part of the family's attempted solution of its problems, and illnesses and feelings in the other members may be part of the patient's effect on his human environment, and therefore of his personality. The illnesses may be seen as not merely disturbances of these individuals' relationships (a point of view as old as psychiatry), but as features of the family as a system. The theory of families as systems, with their subsystems (such as two close children in a family), supra-system (society at large), decider mechanism (such as the dominant parents), and care over outer boundaries, has greatly influenced family therapy, which is often much concerned with networks of power and dominance within the closed system, in which everyone affects everyone else in intense emotional interaction.

The new methods are therefore not just seeing the family together ('conjointly') but using an approach in which the symptoms to be tackled are the pathological systems of .communication in the family (or couple, in marital work). Different approaches are used by different doctors, some conducting sessions using psychodynamic concepts with the individuals of the family, when these seem relevant to motivation; others offering themselves more as teachers and experts in improving methods of communication; some work so exclusively with the 'here-and-now' of the family system that they show little interest in the individuals' uniqueness and do not work towards the acquisition of personal insight by the members of the family; others work mainly by behaviour modification, using contracts and rewards. Co-therapists and even teams are often used.

Sessions are often highly emotional, but the experience has been that they are safe.

There are hardly any results from controlled research: all the enthusiasts agree that change is sometimes remarkably rapid, far more so than with older methods. It may be that the results will also be transient unless accompanied by real change in the individual members. Results are also hard to assess because of difficulty in agreeing on the criteria of success, and one member of the family may get worse as another gets better.

Long intervals are sometimes left between sessions, as continuing repercussions and effects can be assumed when the family go back home after one session to live together until the next. Probably a variety of methods help the members of the family to discover what the other members want from them but have never been able to say, and the therapists often model new forms of behaviour to be copied, especially when they are trying to change the way in which the father or mother behave as a parent.

Most commonly, the parents are encouraged to be in confident control of the children, and a weak father may have to be helped to be more effective and decisive, a change normally welcomed by the entire family.

The indications and contraindications for family therapy are neither clear nor unanimous. Clearly one relevant indication is in families when a child has symptoms of disturbance or a psychosomatic disorder, which is thought, after a diagnostic interview which will often itself be with the whole family, to be connected with marital problems of the parents. The marriage can be discussed in families in front of the children without harm, although sexual matters are still gone into in private sessions. Highly disturbed families with paranoid attitudes and schizoid members are treated together, but not families with one severely ill individual suffering from depression or schizophrenia.

The family therapy movement is accelerating rapidly, and this is not the place to discuss it more fully for students. They can consult Skynner's book and other reading listed at the end of this chapter.

BEHAVIOUR THERAPY

Methods of treatment developed by behaviour therapists have been mentioned in earlier chapters of this book. Examples are token economies for rehabilitating patients with schizophrenia; desensitization and flooding for anxiety and obsessive-compulsive disorders; and the electric buzzer for bedwetting.

Common features essential to the approach are a concentration on clear specification of the items of behaviour to be changed, objective evaluation of progress towards the goal as well as of final results compared with the original baseline, and an eschewing of psychodynamic hypotheses as being unnecessary in the work of treating the patient. Symptom-substitution, predicted by many psychiatrists, has not been found a problem in the work, although this may be partly because of the initial selection of promising patients. The target behaviour is agreed in discussion with the patient, who is expected to cooperate fully in the programme, and will be given tasks of homework to tackle between sessions.

The philosophy is pragmatic as well as scientific, a wide variety of techniques being employed by the controlled, evaluated, but imaginative use of common-sense interventions, and not merely using ideas from experimental psychology. Theory has been left behind, as new treatments are tried by the innovators, and evaluated from the beginning. Classical conditioning as a theoretical basis for some of the methods was succeeded by operant conditioning, and now by modelling, in which the process of learning is speeded up by training the patient to imitate the therapist who demonstrates the desired behaviour. The patient can then be rewarded by praise, or whatever other reward is being employed, for successfully copying the behaviour. This modelling might well be done when training a shy or awkward patient in social skills.

Behaviour covers a wide field for these purposes, so that Lazarus for example, in designing treatment for a patient referred to him for behaviour therapy, will create a multimodal programme with attention to Behaviour, Affect, Sensation, Imagery, Cognition, Interpersonal relations and Drugs. He tweaks the noses of psychoanalysts by his mnemonic for this method: using the above capital letters, he calls it 'Treating the BASIC ID'.

Behaviour therapy has increasingly come to overlap with other forms of psychotherapy, as it emphasizes the importance of a good relationship with the therapist, sees the patient in his social setting, works sometimes in groups and in families, and employs role-playing and games used in encounter groups. Well-conducted, it is no less time-consuming than brief interpretive psychotherapy.

Behaviourally oriented marital therapy has been described especially by Crowe. A behavioural analysis of the marital interactions is made, and discussed with the partners. Usually the deterioration in atmosphere and communication has meant that each is doing and saying very few things that please the other, the encounters being, on the contrary, full of nagging, provocation and hostility. Each partner is then invited to specify, precisely, what improved behaviour he would like to see from the other, and a contract is made, negotiating an exchange of wanted behaviour between the partners. Vague expressions of better attitudes cannot be used; the items have to be specific actions, and of course they often include sexual intercourse. The couple practise the contract at home, scoring behaviour and rewards, until the next session. This principle of 'giving-to-get' although it sounds mechanical, simplistic and demeaning, in practice is not so. Couples often throw themselves with enthusiasm into the contract therapy, the injunctions to ignore upsetting behaviour are a relief, and early results of comparative work show that it is at least as effective as interpretive family therapy in improving marital adjustment.

HYPNOSIS

Hypnosis can be used in supportive and, in certain cases, in interpretive psychotherapy, and in the special application of deconditioning and learning theory in the treatment of phobic states. There are a large number of techniques in existence for the production of complete physical relaxation, leading on to hypnosis of a varying degree. These techniques vary from one operator to another, but the essential principles which most of them have in common include an initial phase of suggestion of relaxation, drowsiness, comfort, and well-being; followed by more specific suggestions of the precise type of hypnotic phenomena which it is desired to produce.

Experience suggests that the best approach is one in which there is a complete absence of tests or challenges of the degree of hypnosis attained, and one in which nothing is promised or even suggested which is not in fact completely within the power of operator and subject together to achieve in the course of any particular session. The detailed practical techniques and possible indications require direct instructions and experience for their mastery. The first edition of this book contained the original working notes for the technique used in the Department of Psychological Medicine of Guy's Hospital. For the reasons contained in the Preface to the Second Edition, these detailed notes have not been retained.

Principal indications for the use of hypnosis
The overall indications for the use of hypnosis in medicine and surgery in general, and psychiatry in particular, are beyond the scope of this account. But valid indications include:

a) States of tension, without depression, but with the autonomic accompaniments of anxiety, or the general adrenergic state (see also (e) below).

b) States in which hypochondriacal symptoms play a large part, again largely in the absence of depression as a primary cause.

c) Allergic and other autonomic effects relating to emotional tension, but of a specific and objectively demonstrable kind e.g. attacks of asthma, migraine, diarrhoea or vomiting, whose incidence can clearly be related at least in some degree to the effects of external stress.

d) Hysterical symptoms which have become habitual, *to the extent that they persist even after thorough investigation and appropriate psychotherapy have elucidated and relieved the psychodynamic situation which precipitated them.*

e) The desensitization technique of behaviour therapy gains when relaxation under hypnosis is substituted for the original technique of Wolpe, which amounted to a direct exhortation to relax, without the powerful and reassuring experience of the subjective diminution of tension experienced in hypnosis to reinforce it. The advantage of the progressive production of relaxation, subjective calmness and confidence, effortless autonomic control, and subsequent well-being induced by hypnosis, is not only that these desirable forms of relief follow smoothly the induction of hypnosis itself, but also that the procedure can be undertaken with all kinds of patients, without risk of harming or alarming them, or complicating their illness in any other way.

Final observations

The overall object of the treatment is simply a reduction of physical tension, leading to an increased control of autonomic function at an unconscious level, and whatever specific benefits may be induced in this way through co-operation of the patient and increase in confidence, morale, and well-being. By the second or third session it should be possible to take the patient straight to the stage of control within five to ten minutes, and concentrate most of the session upon the constructive suggestions which will be used in this stage.

Sessions, other than the first, which will have to include time for the preliminary explanation and reassurance, can usually be limited successfully to half an hour. They may be given once or twice a week, as convenient, or can be given intensively over three or four days per week in certain cases. Where this technique is to be used for the preparation for a relaxed and confident childbirth, in previously anxious and apprehensive patients, six to twelve sessions as an initial course, followed by maintenance sessions once every two or three weeks up to the time of parturition, will prove a sound investment.

The method is designed to achieve the benefit of hypnosis with complete preservation of the doctor/patient relationship on the one hand, and the sensible and honest appreciation of the possibilities of treatment, without magic or mystification, on the other.

Used as a supportive or symptomatic form of psychotherapy, hypnosis can reverse established patterns of hysterical reaction, or conditioned responses involving anxiety or autonomic disturbance, once the underlying psychodynamic basis of these symptoms has been uncovered, and effectively understood and accepted by the patient in preliminary psychotherapeutic interviews. But hypnosis should not be used to abolish symptoms whose psychodynamic basis has not been explored.

In interpretive psychotherapy, the increased rapport can be used to facilitate the recall and re-experience of repressed emotion and to give interpretations an immediate vividness and authority. The disadvantages are that only about one person in five is a suitable subject, and the degree of conscious participation, acceptance, responsibility and full awareness of the emotional implications of the material produced, are all liable to be diminished. This means that it is doubtful whether such a method in which suggestion plays so essential a part can ever be wholly effective in interpretive psychotherapy.

ABREACTION, USING PHYSICAL METHODS

Abreaction is the term given to the explosively rapid release of emotion, in a psychotherapeutic setting. This can occur when previously repressed material is suddenly recalled, whether in normal psychotherapeutic interviews, under hypnosis, or in special circumstances, by the use of physical methods, such as the intravenous injection of solutions of soluble barbiturate preparations or diazepam (Valium). The use of other agents such as ether, or any of the hallucinogenic preparations acting directly upon the cortex, for example cannabis indica and lysergic acid diethylamide (L.S.D.), is no longer generally acceptable.

Abreactive techniques are apt to be particularly valuable when the buried material is comparatively recent and compact, as in the experiences of war, natural catastrophes such as fire, earthquake, avalanche, or other accidents in which the patient may have been involved. Often after such experiences, memory for the event which has been partly or completely lost, can be restored in one or two periods of treatment in which much of the unbearable emotion returns, but is on this occasion accepted and integrated in consciousness.

As well as states of amnesia, recent and severe attacks of acute anxiety will sometimes respond to treatment of this kind. It is obvious that the selection of cases suitable for this type of treatment must be made with great care, and must depend to a considerable extent upon the capacity of the patient to deal with the material released in this heroic fashion. The use of abreactive techniques in patients on the edge of schizophrenic illness, for example, can prove utterly disastrous.

It remains at this point to add that there is some dispute about the degree to which emotional resistance can be overcome by such methods. Certainly in clinical practice, where the well-being of the patient must always take precedence over any and every short cut in treatment, there is little to suggest that patients will disclose under the influence of drugs or anaesthetics, or even under hypnosis, anything which they consciously determined not to disclose before treatment was begun. They may indeed encounter and express memories and ideas of which they were previously *unaware* in consciousness, and which unaided they may be entirely unable to accept or face. But there is no parallel whatever between the use of methods of this kind in the treatment of sick and disturbed people, and those naive misconceptions of their use implied by the term 'truth drug', when applied to them. Information extorted by force or subterfuge against the will of the informant has no place in medicine. Moreover such information is in fact notoriously unreliable, being coloured by the effect of the procedure upon the morale and judgment of the informer, and inevitably influenced in one direction or another by his conception of what his inquisitor wants him to say.

PLANNING TREATMENT

In considering the overall indications for psychiatric treatment in a particular case, the three aetiological considerations originally outlined in Chapter 2 remain useful.

Constitutional and hereditary factors
These represent the most innate and least malleable component of the illness; and, from the patient's point of view, the least explicable: 'But why should this happen to *me*? . . .'

The corresponding therapeutic indication is for an appropriate awareness and recognition of the patient's personal predicament, and acceptance of him as a person in his own right. This is the foundation of the therapeutic relationship. It is absence of such a foundation which so frequently undermines all other therapeutic endeavours.

Environmental exchange
The physiological and psychological exchanges between human beings and their environment play a particularly significant part in the development of psychiatric illness. Therapeutic indications are:

a) Psychotherapy designed to improve the patient's relationship with his environment, and his capacity to understand and deal with it.
b) Appropriate regulation by physical and behavioural treatment of both the degree and the direction of the physical, behavioural, and psychological reaction displayed. In this category come symptomatic treatment, and the specific physiological treatments described.

The personal reaction
The personal experience of illness from the patient's point of view, and his individual psychodynamic response to it, is equally important whether the illness is a mild anxiety state or a severe psychotic reaction such as schizophrenia. Attention to this must be included in psychotherapy, so that the patient's confidence is deservedly won, even before his distress is diminished.

In every case it is part of the doctor's general professional responsibility, after making a diagnosis, to decide first what treatment he can and should undertake himself; and then at what stage (if at all) and for what reason (if any) he should refer the patient for specialist advice or admission to hospital.

An adequate history, a detached but sympathetic acceptance of the patient's initial complaint and predicament, and a combination of appropriate medicinal treatment and supportive psychotherapy, should be within the province of every doctor: whereas the indications for, and the provision of, specialized psychotherapy, or the specific physical techniques in treatment, are decisions reasonably calling for a second opinion. The initial recognition of the existence of serious psychiatric illness, the assessment of the risk of suicide, and the immediate measures appropriate for an emergency remain as always the responsibility of the doctor who first sees the case.

Although in this book physical and psychological methods of treatment have necessarily been described separately, in clinical practice they are essentially complementary; and though in some cases it may be possible to bring relief and even to accelerate recovery by psychological methods alone, it is neither reasonable nor humane to rely upon physical intervention, without individual interest, compassion, and understanding, in the treatment of any patient for any disease.

CONCLUSIONS

In concluding this section on psychotherapy we need to remember its original definition as a method of treatment relying for its effect upon communication between patient and doctor directed towards the relief of the patient's symptoms of distress. This necessarily concise exposition will have made clear that by far the most important factor in effective relief or cure, or indeed change of any kind, is the emotional impact and reality of this kind of communication.

A competent psychiatrist can often see in essence the core of a patient's problems by the time he has completed the preliminary study of the patient's life. Sometimes patients, sensing something of the purpose of this study, will demand an exposition of what is in the doctor's mind, in the belief or hope that this will offer them an immediate key to recovery. But in this sense unfortunately no one can learn from another's experience of his life, no matter how expert or accurate the impression formed by the doctor may prove to be.

We build up our patterns of thought and feeling slowly and often painfully, and the emotional experiences which have gone into them have to be relived rather than retold before we are liberated from their influence upon us. There is all the difference in the world between the intellectual formulation of a man's problems and personality, and that change of heart which alone can bring him release from the chains in which they have bound him. Whether we call the link which the doctor can establish between the one and the other the transference situation or the patient-doctor relationship, we are really dealing with an emotional bond which acts as a catalyst for all the chaotic feeling and experience of the sick or unhappy person.

On the patient's side much of this emotional bond springs, as we have seen, from the reservoirs of stifled and forgotten passions; on the doctor's side from the detached but absolutely sincere and dedicated concern to help, however humbly, another human being. Behind them both there must be that greatest gift of all, a capacity for unselfish love; and for all the wisdom, skill, and technical accomplishment which ought to go into it, psychotherapy is fundamentally but another way of using the creative power of love towards the restoration of human happiness and peace of mind.

In this context one final explanatory fragment of practical clinical advice may be added. It is simply this: the physician confronted by an acutely unhappy, distracted, or suffering patient, must never withhold acceptance, compassion, or understanding; but he must take care how he shows it.

To place a comforting hand on the shoulder of a depressed, schizophrenic, or otherwise psychotic patient may be an act of simple kindness – or occasionally of inspired communication. To do the same to someone in the anguish of neurosis, particularly to someone with hysterical personality, may be to invite misunderstanding, and perhaps to court disaster.

The key to this is simple. Psychotic patients are often like children in a nightmare; whereas neurotic patients are more like disturbed and accusing adolescents, and require a different kind of attention – and respect.

References and Further Reading

Supportive psychotherapy
Chapter XI by D. Stafford-Clark (pp. 277–95), in *Modern trends in psychological medicine – 2*, J. Harding Price (ed.), 1970, London: Butterworths.

Interpretive pychotherapy
Freud: *What Freud really said* by D. Stafford-Clark 1965, Macdonald. Freud, a great writer, can be read in the volumes of the Penguin Freud Library, now appearing. Jung's writings tend to be obscure: he is best approached by way of the Fontana Modern Master *Jung* by Anthony Storr, 1973, and a chapter by I. Champernowne in *Psychotherapy today*, V. Varma (ed.), Constable, 1974. Adler, *The practice and theory of individual psychology*, Routledge and Kegan Paul, 1924.

Historical development
Books by Horney and Fromm are mentioned in the text. For Klein, see H. Segal, *Introduction to the works of Melanie Klein*, Hogarth, 1973. Generally recommended: C. Rycroft's *A critical dictionary of psychoanalysis*, Nelson, 1968. The same author wrote on *Reich*, Fontana, 1971. See also *Freud and the post-Freudians*, by J. A. C. Brown, Penguin, 1961. C. Rogers, *Client-centred therapy* is from Houghton Mifflin, Boston, 1951. *Transactional analysis in psychotherapy*, Grove Press, 1961, describes E. Berne's methods.

For the debate on psychiatry in society, see *American psychiatry, past, present and future*, G. Kriegman et al., University Press of Virginia, 1975.

Brief psychotherapy
See D. H. Malan, *A study of brief psychotherapy*, Tavistock, 1963, and 'The Outcome problem in psychotherapy research', *Archives of General Psychiatry*, 1974, *29*, 719–29.

Therapeutic communities
D. H. Clark, *Administrative therapy – the role of the doctor in the therapeutic community*, Tavistock, 1964; and a classical account of a problem, T. F. Main, 'The Ailment', *British Journal of Medical Psychology*, 1957, *30*, 129–45.

Small group psychotherapy
The clearest accounts for beginners are *The group process as a helping technique* by S. Thompson and J. H. Kahn 1970, Pergamon, and *Small group psychotherapy*, H. Walton (ed.), Penguin, 1971. More advanced is *Group psychotherapy* by S. H. Foulkes and E. J. Anthony, Penguin, 1957. There is an excellent 17-page survey of the present situation in group therapy by R. Skynner in *Psychotherapy today*, V. Varma (ed.), Constable, 1974. Clear thinking, writing and research in a major book are to be found in *The theory and practice of group psychotherapy* by I. D. Yalom, Basic Books, 1970, 2nd edition.

Encounter groups
Encounter groups by C. Rogers, Penguin, 1969, and *Encounter groups: first facts* by M. A. Lieberman et al., Basic Books, 1973.

M. Balint's *The doctor, his patient and the illness*, Pitman, 1957, is essential reading for all doctors.

Family therapy
There is a major English work, *One flesh: separate persons. Principles of family and marital psychotherapy* by A. C. R. Skynner, Constable, 1976, which is readable and comprehensive, with its own reading list. Also *Conjoint family therapy* by V. Satir, Science and Behaviour Books, 1967, and *Marital breakdown: epidemiology and psychotherapy* by S. Crown, a chapter in *Recent advances in clinical psychiatry*, No. 2, edited by K. Granville-Grossman, Churchill-Livingstone, 1976.

Behaviour therapy
'Behavioural psychotherapy' by I. Marks, in *British Journal of Hospital Medicine*, 1976, *15*, 250–6; 'Behavioural treatments in psychiatry', a detailed review by M. J. Crowe, in Granville-Grossman's book (see above) and *Multi-modal behaviour therapy* by A. A. Lazarus, Springer, 1976 (see also p. 137).

Finally, 'A patient's view of psychotherapy', anonymously, in *Lancet*, 1965, *1*, 103.

Chapter 20

Child Psychiatry

INTRODUCTION

The traditional but harmful separation of child psychiatric practice from general psychiatry is at last lessening. The main reasons for this rapprochement are to be found in the increasing interest, among the psychiatrists working with adult patients, in the details of the family interactions which form the setting of the disturbances, but they have yet to realize fully how the interests in joint interviewing of the patient with his relatives, in observation of their effect on each other, in refusing to regard only one member as the obvious patient, and in techniques of family therapy, have been the common coin of the child psychiatrists so long as the profession has existed.

For one special quality of work with the child patient is the inevitability of considering him as a member of his family. He is never in isolation: his behaviour is that of the son who is a worry to his parents, his overactivity is the problem that exhausts his mother, his slowness at school is a disappointment to his academic father, or his brothers and sisters suffer from the way he demands all the available time from both the parents. His feelings will be largely feelings about his family, his own personality is not fully formed, although efforts must be made to reach, understand and help it to develop on its own independent lines, and not merely as is expected of a member of his family. All this is true, and liable to be neglected, in the adult psychiatric patient, yet he, fully grown and adult, can and must also be approached in his own right, with attention paid to his sufferings in his world, and help brought to aid him as an individual in what he wishes to do; in the disturbed small child, on the other hand, the family approach is simply and overwhelmingly the appropriate one.

The other special quality of child psychiatric work is the additional dynamic dimension provided by the fact that the child is developing. He moves on in his increasingly full and complex adaptation to, and participation in the world, so that one prognosis which is sure to be wrong is to say that things will stay the same. The four-year old at home spending the day with his mother, playing games on the carpet in front of the television, may present, when insecure and anxious, with tantrums and refusal to eat, while at six, a schoolboy, he would be more likely to express anxiety by school refusal and clinging to mother.

The principal difficulty peculiar to child psychiatry is of course that the patient is less articulate than the adult in telling the doctor about how he feels, so that the doctor is under greater obligation to collect information from others, to infer the child's mental state from close observation, and to be patient with the child's efforts, first to trust him and then to communicate with him. The doctor will further use additional techniques to help him enter the child's world, from play with toys, in the three and four-year old, to drawing squiggles together in the years following, until the relationship, in the older child, becomes fully realizable in adult discourse.

SERVICES

Psychiatrists and clinics have specialized in treating children for some fifty years now. Child Guidance Clinics, which developed first, have been set up by the educational authority, and tended to deal, to a considerable extent, with referrals from the schools, concerning disturbed behaviour in the classroom, and educational difficulties. Advice was sought on handling at school and possible placement in special facilities, as well as direct treatment for the child. A style of work developed by which a social worker collected background information from the family, and an educational psychologist was available for testing and assessment, especially of intellectual development. School reports would be obtained, and the psychiatrist interviewed the child and the parents. Treatment of the child would usually be a matter for the psychiatrist, while the social worker commonly started case-work with the mother or parents about their side of the family contribution to the genesis of the child's disorder, and their part in the treatment.

Outpatient clinics in child psychiatry are also held as part of the hospital service, and are more accustomed to taking referrals from family doctors and hospital paediatricians. They tend to work in the same general way, but are developing additional services. Admission has rarely been needed, and a few very young disturbed children can be accommodated, if less than satisfactorily, in paediatric wards. But the services have been insufficient, and the principal new developments, long needed, are Day Hospitals for disturbed children (and for their mothers) and admission units for adolescents, usually from 13 to 16.

The residential homes for children, provided by departments of social services, look after many psychiatrically disturbed children among their residents, and those specializing in the disturbed require psychiatric advice for the children and to help and support the staff.

The policy of the Department of Health and Social Security is to form a comprehensive network of child psychiatric services, not so much based on hospitals as they have been heretofore, but with increasing emphasis on community work in home, school and health centre. Consultation, advice, and training for other professions will be at least as important as the clinical treatment provided directly for the patients referred to the staff of the service. A difficult judgment will be required in deciding what proportion of resources to devote to this community work, and what proportion to the traditional clinics.

NORMAL AND ABNORMAL DEVELOPMENT

A synoptic albeit brief view of normal development has already been given in Chapter 3, with especial mention of the importance of the early relationship between mother and infant, and some account of normal psychosexual development is given in Chapter 12.

In the normal child, development proceeds as the result of interaction between the genetic endowment of the individual, as it determines innumerable early and late features of the developing child, and environmental factors, whether physical, psychological or social. Aetiological factors of psychiatric disorder are divided up similarly into these groups.

GENETIC FACTORS

Some illnesses are caused specifically by genetic abnormalities, for example Down's syndrome or mongolism (see Chapter 15).

Sex is determined by the complement of X and Y chromosomes, and apart from the physical differences there are differences in personality detectable early in childhood, before social expectations can be influencing them, and before the children themselves have a concept of 'boy' or 'girl'. In particular boys are from the beginning more active, and are later more aggressive and more prone to tantrums and behaviour disturbances. At these later ages, there is interaction of genetic and environmental factors, in the form of boys' social role which expects them to be in more mischief than girls. Also genetically determined must be the tendency for boys to be over-represented in the extreme and often unhealthy cases of a number of biological phenomena, for example the higher foetal and infantile mortality of boys, and their higher frequency of severe mental handicap and also of very high intelligence at the genius level.

In general, many other factors are sure to be determined by heredity, doubtless more than can be proved at present. That differences of personality are well-marked at birth and continue to develop, is well known to all parents who have had more than one child. Even in this observation, however, environmental factors are not excluded: the infant is seen through the eyes of the mother, whose expectations are different after every birth. She grows older, her life changes, her marriage is not the same, she has different feelings about sons and daughters, and about first and second children, and these feelings affect the way she regards the baby, and the way she reacts to its early behaviour. This reaction in turn then begins to mould the baby's behaviour, and the long process of learning how to react to each other has begun.

The main plan of development is innately determined, a programme coded in the genes, and unfolding through predetermined stages, the sequence of which can scarcely be changed by the environment. The rate of development can be slowed by adverse influences, and when these are removed it may accelerate again, but it cannot be speeded up beyond the rate of the innate process. However, different aspects of development may be relatively forward or behindhand in the course of a general scatter of time-scales for different processes. Intellectual, emotional and physical development may not remain in step, so that for example, severe intellectual handicap, of genetic origin, always accompanied by emotional handicap of greater or less degree, may nevertheless be associated with full physical development (although more commonly this is partially retarded or blemished.) The age of onset of puberty has a wide range of some four years even in normal children.

The development of the personality, if unhindered, thus proceeds at a varying pace, with surges occurring at different times, and with different aspects forging ahead or lagging behind, but all nevertheless part of one movement onwards, like the progress of a flowing tide up an uneven beach.

PHYSICAL FACTORS

The foetus can be injured in pregnancy, as by thalidomide, rubella and probably other viruses, syphilis, and possibly other agents not yet discovered. The new born-infant can certainly be affected biochemically by the mother's state at the time of birth – hypoglycaemia in the case of diabetes, by heroin withdrawal if the mother was dependent on the drug, and by drugs prescribed during labour.

Some cerebral damage caused by birth injury is readily recognized, but minor degrees cause lesser symptoms, such as mild handicaps in motor co-ordination, and this seems to shade off through clumsiness to the normal. It is very likely that minor birth injury has subtle lasting effects on the brain and therefore on personality development, more often than is realized. Other factors handicapping cerebral development, and therefore important in considering the aetiology of mental handicap, are described in Chapter 15.

Any severe physical illness in childhoood may impair emotional and intellectual development at the same time, by a combination of the global effect in holding back all aspects to some extent, although some escape more than others, and the psychological and social effects of prolonged illness, with its pain, disablement, separations from parents and deprivation of education and experience.

PERSONAL AND INTERPERSONAL FACTORS

Separation from the parents, discussed in Chapter 3, although a cause of great distress at the time and for a period afterwards, probably is not a major cause of long-term disorder. It is probable that discordant relationships in the family leading up to the separation have the more lasting effect. Unhappy relationships between the parents, and lack of affection towards the child, are associated with antisocial personality disorders in the child later, and this could arise in more than one way. Failure to form bonds of affection at crucial early stages may damage the ability to form such bonds later, and the development may also be understood in terms of conditioning, by which the child receives cues of disapproval for affectionate behaviour to the parents, and approval for withdrawal and affectionlessness. Alternatively, imitation and modelling of the child on the parent may occur.

In normal development the child's innate capacity is deployed in an environment which encourages the formation of positive responses to people and objects, which stimulates his emerging curiosity, and does not hurt his embryonic emotional reactions. His helplessness and vulnerability need a safe secure atmosphere of affection, acceptance and consistency. Some of his actions are checked and earn disapproval, but these can be set off against the innumerable other occasions when he and his parents are a mutual joy to each other, helping to form a core to his personality in which he feels valuable, wanted and loved.

Over-protection can cause the urge to explore and take risks to wither, and other children and adults may then seem to be awesome, frightening figures. Because innate desires to test independence are thwarted, the child is frustrated, and the seeds of aggression and hostility in the child-parent relationship are sown. The mother's anxiety about the world is readily transmitted to the child, so that there develops a fertile ground for phobias, as well as for physical illnesses, which may be unconsciously encouraged by the mother, if she has hidden motives to keep the child at home with her.

Inconsistency of regime from time to time, or between the two parents or others involved in the upbringing, also leads to anxiety, to faulty learning of social behaviour, or to severe withdrawal from the bewildering situation. If the father encourages adventures like climbing trees, and if the mother is protective when on her own with the child, greatly praising prowess in the field of study, while implicitly denigrating physical activity, what is the child to do when the parents are together, and have no agreed policy?

THE CLINICAL APPROACH

History

The main history of the problem which led to referral is taken from the accompanying parents. The observations made at the time include notes of parental anxiety and attitudes towards the child, their expectations of his development, their hopes when he was born, their comparisons with his brothers and sisters, and their comments on their own childhood. As the parents' personalities were themselves formed in their childhood partially by *their* parents, an account of these people, the patient's grandparents, may be fully relevant to understanding the atmosphere of the family into which he was born. Differences between the parents, or involving one grandparent who lives in the home and has views on upbringing, may become obvious, father or mother seeking the support of the doctor for his or her views about what is the matter with the child.

The initial statement of the presenting problem should be recorded in its exact wording, for this may contain much relevant information, subtly compressed and encoded. There are obvious differences between 'he seems so nervous'; 'he seems so much more nervous than his brother'; 'he seems so nervous and it gets me down'; 'my husband says he seems so nervous'; and 'the other doctor doesn't think he's nervous'. Further questions can be asked to explore the implications of the initial statement and to seek unmentioned problems. Systematic questions can be asked about disturbances of feeding, toilet functions, physical health at different ages, clinging to parents, antisocial behaviour, and behaviour towards brothers and sisters.

The family history of psychiatric disturbances is recorded, as well as themes and personalities found in the family, as described above. Detailed accounts of the development of the other children may throw light on the difficulties experienced with the patient.

A full personal history starts from the mother's physical and emotional health in pregnancy, before reaching an account of the patient's birth. Inquiries are then made after the child's early development, and the ages at which the usual milestones were passed. Separations and other family disturbances are relevant, as well as illnesses, and any other matters that the parents see as having been important in his development. A picture of the developing personality will emerge, with individual interests and patterns of reaction to stress.

After the age of five there may be reports from schools, giving a viewpoint from outside the family on how the child has behaved with other children at play and in formal lessons, in a setting of peers, demands, and discipline.

Examination

The child has to be brought into the consulting room without the parent, and yet without upsetting him or allowing unnecessary opportunity for a demonstration of clinging and inseparability. This is made easier if the clinic and waiting room are none too formal nor forbidding, and show evidence of expecting and understanding children, with toys and comics available. A calm and friendly introduction by the doctor, and an explanation of what he is going to do, can then nearly always be followed by taking the child by the hand and taking him into the consulting room. Over the age of about six, the consultation can be explained in terms comprehensible to the child, with explanation of seeing other children with similar problems and of being keen to help him with his. Fear may be traceable to misconceptions about the visit, apprehension about painful injections, and anticipation that the doctor is sure to be about to advise the parents on punishment for wrong-doing.

Questions can start about name and age, and proceed to likely interests, and questions about school, couched in simple words and on the lookout for apparently compliant answers based on misunderstanding. If subjects that provoke anxiety are approached very gradually, and if necessary obliquely, children will usually talk about their lives and allow inference as to their feelings, although obviously not in adult terms such as 'depression', 'jealousy' and so forth.

A silent and tense child sometimes talks more easily while playing with simple toys such as farmhouse objects and models of family figures, or in trays of sand. Hopes and fantasies may be understood by discussing what his three magic wishes would be, asking about imaginary companions, or joining in tasks of making up stories or drawing pictures.

Physical examination will often be indicated, and may lead to further relevant investigations. Psychological investigations include a standardized assessment of intelligence, using tests of reasoning with older children and in adolescence, but in the smaller children based on such performance as the skill and complexity of drawings.

Assessment and Diagnosis

Consideration of the information as a whole leads to an assessment of the child's capacity and personality, and a formulation of the present problem, expressing how far it is in fact a normal phenomenon, how much it is physical illness, whether it is to be attributed to handicap of intelligence, or whether it can be understood in terms of reaction to stress.

An effort should be made to understand not only what is wrong with the child, but also why he is brought for consultation, now. Is the symptom a meaningless physical phenomenon? Is it an appeal for help, and if so, to whom? Is it a ticket of entry to the doctor? Does this particular symptom have a particular meaning in this family? Does it have nuisance value against the mother or father in a deadlocked situation at home, where there are no direct communications?

CLASSIFICATION

This has always been difficult to make systematic in child psychiatry, as there are few processes that resemble diseases. Most of the patients present with syndromes of disturbed behaviour which need complex formulations in terms of interacting stresses bearing upon the child. A full formulation needs to take account of several dimensions, as in the 'multi-axial classification', recommended by the W.H.O., which reminds us to think of factors in four fields:

1. The clinical psychiatric syndrome – including the disorders of development, of conduct and of personality, neurosis, psychosis, psychosomatic disorders, and the condition of mental handicap as the only significant disorder.

2. A dimension of intelligence,

3. A statement of relevant physical disorders, and

4. A statement of significant psychosocial factors, such as familial problems, parental overcontrol or undercontrol; and deprivation, whether social and material, or of experience, as in children brought up in brutal isolation from the outside world.

PREVALENCE

Figures are available from the research by Rutter and colleagues which screened the whole population of 10-year olds in the Isle of Wight, collecting information from doctors, teachers and the children themselves.

Intellectual and educational retardation of severe degree was found in a total of 8 per cent of the population. This was made up, with considerable overlap between the categories, of 2½ per cent with simple mental handicap, 4 per cent with a specific retardation of reading behind intelligence, and 6 per cent with a general backwardness in reading. Mental handicap was equally common in both sexes, but the specific reading difficulty was much commoner in boys.

Psychiatric disorder sufficiently severe to cause social handicap was found in 7 per cent. Emotional disorders were approximately as common in boys as in girls, while bad behaviour was much commoner in boys. Physical illness was studied at the same time, with a finding that 5½ per cent suffered chronic physical disorder (the commonest conditions were asthma 2·3 per cent of these, epilepsy 0·9 per cent and the group of cerebral palsies and other forms of brain damage, 0·5 per cent).

The total, again with overlap when some children are doubly handicapped or disabled in several ways, is that one child in six, in that socially mixed area, lives with some form of chronic or recurrent handicap. In a poor district of London, at the same time, rates for psychiatric disorder were twice as high, mainly because there were also more unhappy families, mentally ill or criminal parents, sheer poverty and bad schools.

In adolescence at the age of 14, 8 per cent of children stand out as having obvious handicapping psychiatric disorder, but many others, especially emotionally disturbed girls, suffer unknown to the authorities and the services, so that the total is some 21 per cent with psychiatric disorder, slightly more than in childhood.

GENERAL SLOW DEVELOPMENT

This is usually due to the slow maturation of the child who is mentally handicapped, with backward development in all spheres. It is described in Chapter 15.

EDUCATIONAL DIFFICULTIES

These are often caused by unrecognized mental handicap, and will then be largely irremediable. Recognition that the child will always have a mental age below his chronological age can be followed by measures in the schools to reduce the pressure on him, and set realistic expectations in a suitable class.

Emotional problems and unevenness in the process of maturation can also cause educational difficulties, when the child is unready for the education provided for children of his age, or is handicapped by anxiety or behaviour problems. Concentration is poor, or the upsets surrounding his behaviour disrupt his schooling, and he falls behind in educational attainment. Accurate recognition can lead to corrective advice to the parents, support and reassurance for the child, and better educational placement, which may sometimes include remedial coaching or special classes.

DEVELOPMENTAL PROBLEMS OF BEHAVIOUR

Eating difficulties
One of the greatest responsibilities of the mother in charge of her new baby is to be in charge of feeding him: if she does it wrongly he may die. Even toilet training is less of a worry, for the baby will be excreting naturally, and at first the mother is not required to intervene in the process to keep her baby alive. Moreover feeding is nurturing, a part of caring, and a part of loving tenderness. So feeding behaviour is easily disturbed when the relationship between mother and child is an unhappy and strained one, at any age.

In the first year, battles over time-schedules and sufficient amounts can make the baby refuse food and vomit. Habits gradually become set, so that slow eating persists throughout childhood, to the mother's anxiety, frustration and even fury, while on the child's side it is a sign of resistance to the mother, an area of protest in which the mother cannot win. Food fads can arise in this way, but also when the mother is fussily over-protecting the child. Refusal of a new food, an assertion of independence by the child, is followed by a nervous presentation of it by the mother on a later occasion, when the child again refuses. The mother starts regarding him as a nervous child with difficult fads, the child has no incentive to give up the role, and the pattern persists. Any peculiarity of eating can develop in this way, for example vomiting, under-eating, and over-eating. Pica – eating dirt – is one of these, but if it persists to a marked degree beyond the age of three is likely to be a sign of serious illness, especially severe mental handicap.

Nausea and vomiting can also be signs of anxiety or depression by the more direct mechanism of the autonomic disturbances of gastric function associated with these emotions: the child may be sick at any time of stress. Overeating may also arise from the association of intake of food with comfort and satisfaction, so that obesity then results from prolonged excessive food intake assuaging the misery of depression. Obesity may run in the family, for reasons of heredity or, more usually, common habits of overeating among all the members. This in turn may be attributable to the serving of large meals by the housewife, who believes strongly in the importance of all the family 'having enough to eat'. Endocrine causes of obesity must be excluded.

Problems with Sleeping

Battles over getting the child off to sleep, and fearful waking during the night with calls for the parents, are examples of the involvement of sleep in the parent-child relationship, with escalating anxiety and frustration. Disharmony between the parents, with resulting insecurity of the child, may be present, as when the real reason for the child's sleeping in the parental bed is one parent's wish to have a reason for preventing sexual intercourse.

Occasional nightmares and sleepwalking, although alarming at the time, occur in children who need not be regarded as disturbed by more than normal anxieties, and no treatment is required beyond reassurance of the family. Night terrors, and persistence of the other sleep disturbances to a severe degree, may however be symptoms of severe anxiety, and disturbance in the family, and require treatment.

In sleep disorders, simple advice about attitudes, handling and routines may be sufficient. Rarely a hypnotic drug can be prescribed. Closer attention involves detecting the sources of underlying anxiety and conflict, discussing them with the parents and with the child, and sometimes arranging for changes in other stressful situations, for example at school.

Bedwetting

The ages at which children acquire their parents' ability to avoid bedwetting are various, depending in most cases on a ruling factor which is the innate process of maturation of complex patterns of behaviour, but also affected by environmental factors including the parental efforts at training, and emotional problems which disturb the smooth progress of the training process. Few children are dry at night before the age of two. Ten per cent of five-year olds still wet the bed, half that number of ten-year olds, and the proportion continues to fall with increasing age, although a few adults continue to be enuretic most of their lives. These normal figures need to be remembered in the clinical approach to bed-wetting, as an important part is played by the parents' unrealistic expectations of dry beds at an early age, and worries about the child's being abnormal when he is not dry at night by the age of six or seven years.

The common association with a history of persistent bedwetting in a parent, the high frequency of the problem among poor and unintelligent families living in bad conditions, and the prevalence figures mentioned above, all suggest that most persistent bedwetting occurs as an interaction between a pattern of maturation at the slow end of the normal range, and a family environment which is lacking in effective training.

The parents often react with hostility and resentment, and the helpless child becomes terrified of their response to his next wet bed, the resulting family friction inhibiting further successful training. The child's bedwetting can have started as a disturbed emotional response to the family situation, even as revenge on the mother, but this is much less common than the situation when the emotional disturbance in the child comes later, in response to the misery of being unable to stop bedwetting.

Certainly bedwetting is sometimes a symptom of widespread emotional disturbance, but when this is the case other disturbances and neurotic symptoms will be in evidence. When the bedwetting is of late onset after a substantial period of achievement of dry nights, it may represent a regressive reaction to the stress of anxiety or depression, and investigation of this possibility needs to be more thoroughgoing.

Physical causes, often suspected, are in fact rare. The history may lead to suspicion of abnormalities of the urinary tract, or of spinal reflex control, if there have been incontinence by day or urinary infections. Epilepsy is a possible cause of bedwetting. If there is no suggestion of physical abnormality from the history or physical examination, extensive specialist investigations are not normally needed except for testing of the urine, and they are upsetting to the child.

Treatment starts with the consultation itself, in which the pressure is taken off the child. Calm discussion with child and parents about how many children of that age suffer from the problem, but will not do so permanently, soothes the atmosphere, and can be followed by advice to the parents about rewards and attention for dry nights, with a total suspension of criticism for the wet ones. A chart is given to the child and explained to him. It is not sufficient to end by assuring that 'he will grow out of it': he may not grow out of it for some time, and resentment will continue unless the parents cease to worry about the child's excretory progress, which is unlikely.

The child needs to be seen again to hear of progress, look at his chart of wet and dry nights, and praise the dry nights enthusiastically. The next treatment is with the drug imipramine in a dose initially of 25 mg at bedtime, but with the possibility of increasing to 50 mg or occasionally more in older children. The mechanism of action is unknown, but if the drug is combined with frequent reviews of progress and checks that the attitude of the family to wet beds is improving, excellent results are obtained, with rapid progress to full dryness in about three-quarters of cases. When the drug is withdrawn, however, many relapses occur. These relapses in their turn are reviewed to assess whether the stage of maturation is not yet equal to reliable bladder control at night, or whether adverse circumstances are hampering the child's progress.

N.B. Beware of the dangers of tablets in a house with young children – imipramine in accidental overdosage is highly dangerous.

The children are often reported by the parents to be very deep sleepers, and prescription of amphetamine in small doses sometimes can alleviate this, with consequent easier awakening in response to the full bladder.

The electrically operated alarm buzzer, triggered by the first drops of urine dampening pads between the sheets, has in careful hands obtained the best results, over 80 per cent of cases being cured. The method can be tried in most children from the age of six upwards. Very detailed instructions need to be followed, to ensure that the alarm operates as promptly as possible, and is loud enough to wake the child at once. The child gets up to stop the buzzer and empty his bladder, and the bed has to be attended to. There is often a period of difficulty in making the apparatus work, and the family need to persist patiently for several months, as well as having the chance to report their problems during this time. The buzzers are commercially available, or they can be hired from many clinics.

It is always assumed that this treatment works by a conditioning process, training a reflex that was not present before, linking micturition and wakening, but the theory is not satisfactory, and the treatment is likely to work in a number of ways.

Encopresis

After the age of two years, soiling with faeces becomes rare, and when it is persistent, and not due to physical disorder, it is usually a sign of severe psychiatric disturbance. The child is usually under great stress when brought to the doctor, and is often being punished severely. Psychological treatment directed to the emotional disturbance of the child and family is required.

PROBLEMS OF SEXUAL BEHAVIOUR

Masturbation can be found at all ages, from primitive manipulation of the genitals in the first two years of life, to increasingly complex and erotic behaviour with sexual fantasies, in later childhood. In adolescence it is universal in boys, and found in the majority of girls; it is therefore normal in both sexes. Parental concern may be based on ignorance of this, and on strong feelings about sexual matters, which may be susceptible to discussion with the doctor. Masturbation is itself a sign of something amiss only when it becomes extremely frequent and is used compulsively to relieve tension. These children are often lonely, bored, and anxious, as well as guilty about the masturbation.

Homosexual behaviour and *sexual deviations* may be noticed in early forms in childhood: they are referred to in Chapter 12.

Sexual promiscuity has usually been noticed as a feature of delinquent children who break many social rules and form few lasting relationships. The mores of the social setting are changing, however, and doubtless more promiscuity in relatively normal young people will be seen.

Victims of sexual assaults may need to be examined. Some of these children seem to be hardly disturbed by the event, but some are severely frightened and guilty afterwards, although this is sometimes hidden. The victims may be repeatedly involved in incidents of similar type, and may be helping, by seductive behaviour, to precipitate or at least not to terminate, the incidents. Parental horror and preoccupation may do far more harm than the incident itself and the police inquiries, and time taken with the parents to persuade them to allow the incident to be forgotten, is well spent.

Child victims of father-daughter *incest*, also, may be seductive and collude with the relationship over long periods, as does sometimes the mother. The girl is not necessarily gravely disturbed afterwards, although support will be needed during an inevitable period of family strife after the exposure.

PROBLEMS OVER ATTENDANCE AT SCHOOL

Truancy is delinquent, *school phobia* is neurotic. The truant is usually showing other anti-social traits, described below, and is bored at school as well as doing badly at schoolwork. He is deceitful about the non-attendance and is not anxious. The attitude of the parents has often been indifference, neglect or hostility; rarely is the family a happy and caring one. Truants with disturbed personalities may spend the day in solitary and sometimes anti-social activities out of school. Wider social factors are also of great importance in understanding truancy, which becomes more frequent when schools are poor, the school-leaving age is raised, and local gangs assemble to plan exciting forays.

The child with school phobia, on the other hand, has anxieties over leaving home and mother, who is usually herself anxiously overprotective, as well as being lonely, and motivated to keep the child with her. Anxiety is readily provoked by the approach of the separation for the journey to school, where the child has frequently done well as a model well-behaved pupil. Crises of school refusal occur typically at times of family stress, when the child dreads breakup of the home or loss of the parents while he is absent, or when he has to face a new school. Treatment involves exploring, understanding, interpreting, and if possible changing the emotional disorders in the family relationships. The difficulty is to combine the necessarily slow tempo of psychotherapy with the urgent need for firm insistence on return to school, for education may be endangered for many months, and the longer the period away from school, the harder it will be to break the pattern. The threat of legal sanctions may be needed, as well as tranquillizing drugs.

DELINQUENCY

This is used here as a convenient heading for the children who break legal or moral and customary rules, who may be brought to see doctors in consequence.

Isolated incidents of truancy, small thefts, vandalism, wandering away, lying or cruelty are normal events in virtually all children, as they test the limits of what is allowed, try the experience of naughtiness and guilt, and observe their parents' reaction. The timid and conscientious make the smallest of ventures; the bold, assertive and selfcentred transgress more often, and in ways which cannot be so easily ignored.

Persistent delinquency is partially a passing phenomenon of later childhood and adolescence, but also in many cases is continuous with the same behaviour in later life. The problems of crime, not in itself a field of psychiatry, and of psychopathic personality, are discussed in Chapter 11.

The children as a group have a spread of intelligence close to the average, although they are often undereducated in relation to their ability. Physically they tend to be athletic and active. Their family backgrounds contain many broken families, neglectful and rejecting parents. Family traditions of connivance at law-breaking and irresponsible behaviour merge into the effect of growing up in areas where the anti-social culture is a powerful influence. More widely, the social causes of delinquency are the predominant ones. These may include poverty and poor housing in disorganized cities where respect for fellow-humanity is hard to achieve; the disparity between the advocacy of materialist affluence and what goods are legitimately available to the poor; the aggressive and sexual drives of adolescents in conditions of crowding and breakdown of traditional forms of parental, religious and legal authority; and other related hypotheses.

The ages at which antisocial behaviour is a common problem are from 10 onwards through adolescence to a falling-off in early adult life. For actual crimes the peak age is around thirteen. In the criminal statistics lawbreaking is far commoner in boys than girls, but the rule-breaking of the girls includes promiscuity, disapproved of by society but not counted in the figures. Many of the crimes are committed in gangs or very small groups of two or three associates, a typical phenomenon of adolescence.

Much of the delinquency of late childhood and adolescence is thus to be understood in a social context, the individuals being psychiatrically normal. It is a pursuit of excessive masculinity and femininity; testing the limits, under pressures from peer-group and society at large, at the uneasy time of puberty; experimenting with being nearly adult.

The problem of disturbed anti-social individuals remains, however, within the wider phenomenon. Adult *psychopathic personalities* can be traced back to the age of five to six, when much of personality, including commitment to moral and social values, has been formed. Persistent stealing is common, originally from parents, but spreading to school and elsewhere. The pattern is readily understandable in terms of the disturbance of the ability of the child to have affectionate bonds with those around him: he steals symbolic value from his parents, and tests their reaction. He may use the money to buy superficial regard from other children, having no close friends of his own. Persistent cruelty to other children and animals, and marked aggressive traits, are also signs of severe disturbance of personality.

The superficial pleasure-seeking often appears to be joyless, may be symbolic (as in the above example of taking valuables from the parents) and can be motivated by the desire to elicit a response from the parents. This is sometimes in the form of repeatedly having to rescue the child from the retribution of others, but may be harshly condemnatory. The child learns to deal with his unhappiness by convincing himself that he does not care, and develops the outward appearance of a hard-bitten outcast from society. It has been said that psychopathic personalities are not so much unable to form relationships, as crippled by unresolved bitter relationships with parents in the past.

Treatment is attempted in the psychiatrically disturbed individuals. Forms of supervision and training are needed, by probation officers and social workers, with a variety of institutional measures. There are schools for maladjusted children, on a day basis or for boarders, and children's homes for those in the care of the local authority. Inpatient hospital units and day hospitals increasingly employ group psychotherapeutic methods as well as educational and training skills, and high numbers of specialized staff. The prognosis for short-term change in severely antisocial young people nevertheless remains poor.

BODILY MOVEMENTS AND HABITS

Hyperkinesis is a syndrome which may appear at age 1–4 and usually improves greatly later in childhood, troublesome cases being rare after the age of 10. The restless activity, exploration, distractibility and sometimes aggressiveness of these children leads to exhaustion of the family, with increasing rejection, and identification as a problem, which they are. Their education is greatly hampered. Unceasing movement, clumsiness and upsets with other children in the class may lead to exclusion from school, and further handicap in learning.

In some cases there are neurological syndromes or generalized mild brain damage, as well as degrees of intellectual handicap. The increased frequency of a history and signs of dysfunction of the central nervous system in a series of these children strongly suggests that minimal brain damage is the critical cause of the syndrome in perhaps the majority. Epilepsy is one of the associated conditions in some cases, and E.E.G. investigation may be indicated.

Nevertheless some cases appear to be of emotional origin, anxiety or frustration having led to bodily overactivity, to which parents, siblings, and staff at school reacted. A vicious circle is liable to occur in all cases, including those with undoubted organic handicap. The overactive behaviour ensures that the child is an unwelcome problem and has difficulty in concentrating and learning. Parents and school attempt control and punishment, to his increasing distress, which is then manifest in greater hyperkinesis.

Treatment is with a combination of psychotherapy, designed to relieve the emotional complications, and medication, based either on haloperidol, in experimentally increasing doses, or on the paradoxical sedative action of methylphenidate (20–80 mg daily) or dexamphetamine (10–40 mg daily).

Tics or habit spasms, repeated stereotyped jerky movements, especially of parts of the face and neck, are common complaints in children. Sometimes the child coughs and grunts at the same time. Most commonly the cause is never elucidated, although disturbed patterns of emotion and attention in the family are often suspected, and occasionally an interpretation in terms of body-language is convincing. (Shakes of the head, for example, may be fragmentary negative gestures.) Most tics disappear spontaneously after a harmless course of some months or a year or two, but sometimes psychotherapeutic attention to the family is needed: discussion of patterns of attention and reward, with the child keeping his own charts of severity.

Gilles de la Tourette's syndrome is the name given to the condition when the meaningless grunts become fragmentary ejaculations of words, especially obscenities. There are subtle signs of minimal cerebral dysfunction in many of these children, and haloperidol has been as effective a treatment as any others that have been tried.

Nail-biting is common, declining in frequency with age but sometimes persisting into adult life as a minor habit. The children are sometimes but not always notably tense. They regard the symptoms as being under their ultimate control, and attempts at treatment are unrewarding.

Head-banging and rocking up to the age of about three, are sometimes associated with mental handicap, but also occur as habits in perfectly normal children, when they usually require no treatment.

DISORDERS OF DEVELOPMENT OF SPEECH

Stammering occurs in about 4 per cent of children at some time, and is found in about 1 per cent at any one time, much more commonly in boys and slightly more commonly in those of low intelligence. The causes are unknown, the theories of heredity, incomplete cerebral dominance, and emotional maladjustment in the field of choking back aggression, all being unsupported by good evidence.

Many transient and mild stammerers slowly become fluent as they grow older, but those with the more severe disability fail to do so, and still stammer in adult life. These individuals may suffer emotional maladjustment as a result of the social disability of the stammering itself.

Severe stammering is treated by speech therapists by a variety of techniques, including practising rhythmic speech, delayed feedback of the subjects' own speech through earphones, and behaviour therapy with desensitization to situations liable to provoke the worst stammering. Counselling the parents about their handling of the disability is required, and sometimes the treatment of the child himself has considerable psychotherapeutic content.

Delayed speech is a very important problem in diagnosis. It may be caused by mental handicap, brain damage, deafness or psychosis, and is sometimes an elective mutism in the setting of a disturbed relationship between mother and child.

Dyslexia, disability in reading, occurs in the general form with other features of delayed maturation, but also in a specific relatively isolated syndrome. These children may often be left-handed and have associated difficulties with speech, which suggest that the disability may be attributable to a subtle parietal lobe lesion, but this is far from certain. Remedial teaching in reading is long and arduous.

TEMPER TANTRUMS

The pre-school child's behaviour may become dominated, in the eyes of his family, by aggressive acts of temper, defiance and refusal of the parents' requests to behave. The child's fighting back for control and domination of his world knows no bounds, as in Bentovim's vivid illustration quoted in full:

'A boy was seen aged 3 years 8 months who had been becoming increasingly difficult over six months. Severe violent temper tantrums were the main complaint, often set off without obvious reason but sometimes provoked by minor frustrations. He had to have the last word, would shout "No" to any request, hurl objects around, smashing many of his toys, and demand the television at any time, even learning to plug it in himself. His parents had tried every way of stopping him, putting him in his room, but he showed a tremendous amount of strength. There was no evidence of any medical cause such as temporal lobe epilepsy. Sometimes he could be pacified and talked out of an attack but generally it was impossible to stop him.

He had always been a temperamentally difficult boy – on the go with considerable intensity of play. His development had been rapid, but he could only be got to sleep by being driven around the block in the early days. He was a finicky feeder and was very reluctant to chew – the only area he failed to "bite on" whole-heartedly. His controlling, disobedient, violent behaviour was limited to the home and did not occur in nursery school.

There were no obvious precipitating factors to his gradually increasing temper outbursts. Seeing the family together in a conjoint family interview, however, did offer some clues. His own pattern of play indicated a preoccupation with battles. His mother's angry posture, tone, and general attitude towards her son indicated that she was as angry herself. It appeared that she was provoked and was in turn provoking. Their battles seemed endless. She described her brother as having had similar behaviour with her own parents. The father, a rather more placid and controlled person but with a considerable temper when roused, seemed less concerned in the friction. Indeed, he had been able to stand back and observe the way the family behaved even before the consultation. He had realised that his son was almost deliberately going out of his way to irritate them, appearing to give himself a reason to have the tantrum, as if to say "Now you've been angry with me, I can be angry with you, even if I started it". The father encouraged his wife to ignore this behaviour, and when there was a severe tantrum his father together with a friend had held him firmly for an hour. They held on until he calmed down. On that occasion he could not convince himself that he really did have bad parents who were cruel and angry, making it safe for him to bully at whatever cost. He emerged from this tantrum in a far more friendly mood, and began to be affectionate and loving in a way that his parents had not experienced before. He also suddenly began to talk about events such as his sister's birth which he had not acknowledged previously. The doctor's task in this case was to help them understand what they had enacted spontaneously.'

NEUROTIC SYMPTOMS

Anxiety and phobias

Anxiety tends to be manifest, especially from the age of five onwards, in muscular tension, fearfulness, and phobic avoidance of particular situations or objects. The fears may be adopted from the fearful overprotective mother, for instance, when she explains her own terror of spiders, thunderstorms, or men hiding in the shadows in the streets at night. Single frightening experiences may lead to learning of a phobia, and consistent avoidance of the feared situation afterwards means that the fear is never tested in reality and given the chance to be extinguished.

Common fears are of the illness or death of the mother, father, brothers or sisters, and in these cases the child's ambivalent feelings of love and hate may be detectable, as well as the setting of anxious insecurity in the family, and stress bearing upon the child in particular. Examples of threatening situations include problems in family life (drunkard father, depressed mother, handicapped sibling) or at school (academic pressure to which the child is not equal, bullying, racial prejudice, etc.). Older children may fear that they themselves will die or be afflicted by terrible illnesses. School phobia and its typical background have been described above, and so has the association of night terrors with anxiety.

Obsessive-compulsive symptoms

Obsessive-compulsive symptoms, especially rituals, are common, nearly always as transient phenomena. They originate in magical ways of coping with and neutralizing anxiety, but then may persist as conditioned habits after the meaning has drained from them.

The mechanisms are the same as those described in Chapter 10, but can more easily be studied in children.

Treatment is by psychotherapy or behaviour therapy, and sometimes by additional prescriptions of tranquillizing drugs in the short term.

DEPRESSION

In the sense of severe unhappiness which impairs health and normal life, forms of depression are detectable from infancy, when the child separated from the mother fails to thrive (see Chapter 3). Later in childhood, depression may be the underlying reason for antisocial behaviour, failure to learn at school, regression to earlier forms of behaviour (for example: bedwetting), and general ill-health. Illnesses resembling the psychotic depressions of adults and not obviously related to life events are very rare, as is suicide before the age of fifteen.

Treatment is usually directed at relieving the unhappiness, but tricyclic antidepressant drugs are also valuable, in doses appropriate to the size of the child.

PSYCHOSIS

Early infantile autism or psychosis

This condition starts usually within the first year, and certainly before the age of three. It is rare, with an incidence of 4·5 per 10,000 children. It is commoner in boys than in girls, and in families with parents in high social classes.

The children are often thought to have been always hard 'to get through to' and unresponsive to cuddling. The characteristic behaviour of the psychosis is

1 profound social withdrawal from gaze, touch and social involvement,
2 the child is mute, or severely handicapped by fragmentary and bizarre speech, odd use of pronouns, and other idiosyncracies,
3 tenacious rituals ensuring concentration on sameness in the child's environment, with catastrophic emotional reactions to change,
4 other odd postures, grimaces and habits.

Intelligence is hard to test, but is usually handicapped, often to below I.Q. 60, although the behaviour described above is different from that of other mentally handicapped children. The odd, withdrawn behaviour, gross handicap in speech, and tendency to wander around make psychotic children ineducable in ordinary schools.

The cause is unknown. There is no tendency to have a family history of schizophrenia, nor other evidence of heredity. Early suggestions that the parents were aloof, cold and academically demanding have not been confirmed, but there are, increasingly, pieces of evidence pointing to a variety of subtle forms of cerebral dysfunction in up to 50 per cent of cases. The explanation for the syndrome could then be that the children have a receptive dysphasia, and cannot comprehend sounds. Their relatively intelligent and verbally fluent parents unwittingly bombard them with language, and the children over-react in a complex syndrome of withdrawal, inability to comprehend, and disruption of what little speech they acquire.

Differential diagnosis is from deafness, ordinary mental handicap, extreme emotional stress in very eccentric children, rare cerebral disorders, and late psychosis of childhood.

Treatment is by educational and training approaches to the children, especially using touch and movement, by affectionate nurses, and requiring most unusual gifts of patience and persistence. Operant conditioning of social skills is partially successful, but the gains rapidly decay when the enthusiasm of the programme diminishes, so that the parents must be taught the training techniques, too. Much support and advice is needed by the parents throughout.

The prognosis for the future of the children is very poor; most stay in institutions, growing up to be autistic and handicapped adults. Barely a tenth – those with some speech and not severely handicapped in intelligence – make some social adjustment to life outside hospital. Phenothiazine drugs do not change the process but may help to control behaviour.

Late infantile psychosis or childhood schizophrenia
From the age of eight onwards, rare cases of schizophrenia occur. Hallucinations, delusions and feelings of passivity of thinking occur, as in adults, and there is often a family history of schizophrenia. Organic illness must be excluded, and treatment then depends on phenothiazine drugs and supportive psychotherapeutic measures for the family. Schizophrenia is described fully in Chapter 6.

CEREBRAL DISORDERS

Acute delirious states, with distractibility, clouding of consciousness, and visual hallucinations, are common in children, and are usually transient.

Brain damage may arise in numerous ways, including inherited cerebral abnormalities, pre-natal damage from harmful influences on the foetus, and environmental causes during childhood. The latter include birth injury, neonatal jaundice, encephalitis, the sequelae of epileptic fits, and head injury in accidents.

The psychiatric disorder in the child has two major aspects: a) the handicap itself, including often an epileptic handicap, and of course any focal signs of neurological deficit, and b) the reaction to this, in the child and in those around him.

The cerebral disorder hampers general development and intelligence, by damaging the capacity to learn, and by delaying the emergence of specific skills and motor coordination. Typical features in the behaviour of the brain-damaged child, as well as the usual low intelligence, are distractibility, because of the short attention-span, and hyperkinesis. There are also often difficulties with labile and intense moods, which are commonly aggressive tantrums but also may be episodes of anxiety. In children with the onset of brain damage during childhood, it can be seen that these symptoms are a marked coarsening of pre-existing features of the child's developing personality.

The nature of the child's response to his disability, and equally the response of parents and school, plays a profound part in influencing the course of the disorder. The child with minor degrees of damage, and average intelligence, may be regarded by his parents and teachers as very slow to develop, lazy and difficult. He is then rejected and punished. He tends to react by frustration, anger and anxiety, which may increase his hyperactivity and inability to concentrate and learn.

Investigation requires a particularly careful history of illnesses and of the stages of development, followed by a physical examination with a vigilant search for neurological signs. Tests of motor coordination and of ability to concentrate must be included. Psychological testing appropriate for the age may be helpful for fuller analysis of intellectual function, and to establish a baseline from which to study further progress. The electroencephalograph is rarely a crucial investigation, because of the high proportion of 'immature' tracings, with slow waves, found in normal children, and because hardly any tracing is pathognomonic of diffuse brain damage.

Treatment may use drugs for the control of hyperkinesis (described above), but the principal help need is psychotherapeutic, in the form of discussing family attitudes to the child, and endeavouring to relieve the emotional difficulties arising from the disability, and from how it is handled by those around him.

Epilepsy is common, being found in nearly 1 per cent of ten-year-old children in the Isle of Wight survey. The causes are similar to the causes of brain damage just described, with a hereditary element, presumably a constitutional low threshold of firing into a fit, and with an additional cause being febrile convulsions. Contrary to earlier beliefs, these are not harmless, and probably often lead to minimal degrees of brain damage, especially if a number of fits occur in quick succession. The different types of fit will not be described in this textbook of psychiatry. The psychiatric disturbances of epileptics, much more frequent than in the physically handicapped children, include the low intelligence, on average, and non-ictal episodic disturbances, especially great overactivity, or violent rages (typically when the lesion is in the temporal lobe). However, many of the difficulties typical of epileptic children, such as underachieving at school, are caused by many interacting factors between the specific epileptic handicap of the brain, the low intelligence, and the reaction of the child and parents to the epilepsy, its meaning, its difficulties and its stigma. The parents, the school, and others are often much more frightened by the first fits than is realized, and their attitude to the child may become markedly overprotective, or the opposite, rejecting.

Treatment consists of anti-convulsant medication plus at least as close attention to psychological and social measures, to relieve these additional difficulties, whether they pre-date or post-date the fits themselves.

TREATMENT

The traditional psychotherapeutic approach, basically derived from psychoanalysis, but modified for children and adapted for use in shorter periods of treatment, is becoming a less predominant mode. The clinics were able to offer treatment, as distinct from assessment and reports, for too few patients, after long periods of waiting.

Increasing criticism of this approach, and realization that there is little evidence that psychotherapy of this type is effective, have led to many changes of style, especially in the last fifteen years.

Briefer treatment and simple counselling have been tried, with more concentration on limited goals, such as the removal of a few named target symptoms or problems. Increasingly, the family are seen together for what is explicitly family therapy, and the father is required as much as the mother. With greater scepticism and humility about good results, these shorter periods of treatment have been offered from the beginning, sometimes combined with a specific contract stating this to the family.

At the same time, as part of the movement of innovation and giving high priority to scientific approaches which encourage evaluation, the place of behavioural methods has grown. They have been used for the desensitization of phobias, although the technique is more difficult than with adults. The (incompletely understood) success of the buzzer-conditioner in the treatment of bedwetting has already been mentioned. Early experiments in the application of these methods to disruptive behaviour in the classroom and at home have also been encouraging: teachers or parents are trained in systematically ignoring the unwanted behaviour while encouraging better behaviour by attention, praise and other rewards.

The movement towards consultations with other people in contact with disturbed children involves discussions with staff of children's homes and schools, especially remedial classes, as well as families in the home. Professional roles become blurred, and much more treatment is being given by trained social workers, and very recently, nurses. The training of nurses to be skilled in psychotherapy and behaviour therapy is only beginning, but will certainly become increasingly important, and they will then be able to join the team of consultants and therapists in the clinic or with other agencies.

References and Further Reading

Maternal deprivation reassessed by M. Rutter, 1972, Harmondsworth: Penguin, reviews the subject clearly.

The multi-axial system of classification is described in *Psychological Medicine* 1973, *3*, 244–50.

The Isle of Wight studies are discussed in full in *Education, health and behaviour*, M. Rutter, J. Tizard and K. Whitmore,

1972, London: Longman, and summarized in *Psychological Medicine* 1976, *6*, 313–32.

A. Bentovim's case is in his excellent article in *British Medical Journal* 1976, *1*, 947–9: 'Disobedience and violent behaviour in children: family pathology and family treatment'.

Autism can be studied in *Early childhood autism*, edited by Lorna Wing, 1976, Oxford: Pergamon.

A review of the psychiatry of adolescence is found in an article of that title in *British Journal of Hospital Medicine* 1976, *16*, 575–82, by S. N. Wolkind and J. C. Coleman.

'Stuttering: some Facts and Treatments' is a review by F. Fransella in *British Journal of Hospital Medicine* 1976, *16*, 70–7.

Services are described by D. M. Scott et al. in Chapter 10 of *Comprehensive psychiatric care*, edited by A. A. Baker, 1976, Oxford: Blackwell, and developments in treatment are rapidly reviewed by P. Graham, 'Management in child psychiatry: recent trends', in *British Journal of Psychiatry* 1976, *129*, 97–108. There is an excellent chapter, with 297 references, by I. Kolvin and A. Macmillan, in *Recent Advances in Clinical Psychiatry, Number 2*, edited by K. Granville-Grossman 1976, Edinburgh: Churchill-Livingstone, pp. 296–350.

Also recommended: *Childhood disorder – a psychosomatic approach*, by P. Pinkerton, 1974, Crosby, Lockwood, Staples (very good on clinical accounts of families); and *Helping troubled children*, by M. Rutter, 1975, Harmondsworth: Penguin, for a lucid account written for the non-specialist. A general textbook is *Basic child psychiatry* by Philip Barker, 1971, London: Staples.

A Personal Reflection
From Author to Reader

Human suffering is inevitably complex. Its complexity has always required that doctors be trained to deal with unhappiness and fear as well as with pain: with defensive shyness or reserve, as well as with the physical guarding of tense muscles over a tender spot. They need to learn that brusqueness can be as cruel as clumsy handling of damaged tissues, and that the relationship between doctor and patient demands as much forbearance, imagination and unselfishness as that between parent and child. Yet they cannot be expected to gain this necessary wisdom from the precept or example, still all too prevalent, which leads them to regard the diagnosis of neuroses in patients complaining of physical symptoms as tantamount to the unmasking of an impostor – a process of scientific deduction which may bring credit and satisfaction to the doctor, but which is chiefly valuable in relieving him of any further responsibility towards the patient so skilfully discredited. What then is the contribution of psychiatry to this problem?

I think the text of its message, of the precepts which psychiatry must hold and the example which psychiatry must set, can best be summed up in a memorable line from Arthur Miller's play, *Death of a salesman*. The words are spoken by the wife of the doomed man, when she is attempting to awaken the conscience, compassion and humanity of her two sons towards the father who has endlessly indulged them but whom they now affect to despise. They have discovered his pathetic and sordid preparations for suicide – and their reaction is simply to recoil in horror. Projecting some of their guilt as hostility towards this man whom they can see only as a source of worry to the mother on whom they still depend, they wax indignant about his cowardice and underhandedness in thus sneaking off ignobly to die, leaving all his problems still unsolved. Their mother, suddenly become wise and eloquent in her comprehension of the ultimate tragedy of the situation, rounds on them fiercely, reminding them both of their relationship to their father, of his need of them and of her, and of his search for an understanding which he has never achieved – either from most of the people with whom he has dealt, or of himself and within his own heart. 'Attention', she says, 'attention must finally be paid to such a person. . . .'

This above all seems to me to be the key to the practice of medicine and surgery as well as to the practice of psychiatry; the key to the contribution which psychiatry has to make, and to the values which it enshrines. Attention must be paid to the individual man and woman, no matter what the nature of their sickness or suffering, no matter how severe the disturbance or distortion of their world or their contact with others, no matter how strange or even frightening they may appear, no matter how sordid or ignominious their predicament. In the special context of the phrase 'attention' means, not simply interest, not even simply compassion, but the active, dedicated, detached, but uncompromising love for other human beings which alone can inspire and ultimately crown the highest endeavours of medicine.

The contribution of psychiatry to a fuller understanding of the principles and practice of medicine must ultimately be to underline a single fundamental truth: the essential wholeness and dignity of man. For although the technique of psychiatry as part of the training of a medical student is of great importance throughout the entire complicated field of human relationship, and of mental health and sickness, it is in this bridge between what are commonly regarded as essentially medical, surgical, gynaecological or obstetric disorders, and their emotional aspects and manifestations, that the whole truth of medicine begins best to be understood.

Confronted by any sick, frightened, disturbed or unhappy person, the doctor can always remember this simple precept: 'Attention must be paid to such a person . . .' Once a patient realizes that you care about how he feels, then you have given him a bridge, to link his need to your capacity to help him, a bridge which he can cross to meet you and which you can cross to meet him. Good doctors have always recognized the necessity for such a bridge: the best have discovered something of the way to build it for themselves and their patients. In this sense the better the doctor, the fuller will be his recognition of his own need for psychiatric knowledge and skill; and the more complete his attainment of these objectives, the better doctor will he yet become.

D. S.-C.

Questions for Revision, Reflection and Discussion

Chapter 1

What is the field of psychiatry?

How do patients, other people, and doctors react to physical and to psychiatric illness?

Chapter 2

What information should be recorded in a full psychiatric history? How is it to be elicited, and under what headings?

What headings are used for recording the mental state of the patient? Which abnormalities are recorded under the headings?

How is intelligence distributed in the population? What is the significance of the figures in everyday life?

Chapter 3

How does a baby develop awareness of itself as an individual? How does the relationship with the mother develop? How do children react to separation from their mother?

Describe the psychology of adolescence.

What are the differences between senile dementia and normal old age?

Describe the psychodynamic hypothesis, including the concepts of repression and the unconscious.

Chapter 4

How are psychiatric disorders classified?

Chapter 5

What conditions lead to acute confusional states?
What are the clinical features of the state?
What are the psychiatric effects of epilepsy?
What are the clinical features of dementia? How is it diagnosed
and investigated? What are the methods of management and
treatment?

Chapter 6

Discuss the aetiology of schizophrenia, distinguishing suggestions
from facts. What are the clinical features? Explain the technical terms you use in the description. How is the illness treated?
With what results?

Chapter 7

What are the causes of depression? What are the clinical features?
Compare them with a description of mania. Explain the terms
sometimes used in classifying depressions.
Discuss suicide rates in detail. Compare the demography and
psychiatry of suicide and attempted suicide.
Describe grief after bereavement, and how it can be helped.
How is depression treated?

Chapter 8

Discuss the aetiology of, and ways of regarding, anxiety. What
clinical syndromes occur? What methods of treatment are used?
When the main features are phobias, how are they treated?

Chapter 9

How are hysterical illnesses best defined? Explain the stresses and
other factors involved in the development of hysterical syndromes.
What determines which function is incapacitated? What is the
treatment?

Chapter 10

Define obsessive-compulsive phenomena. How are they to be understood? How can distressing symptoms be treated?

Chapter 11

Describe psychopathic personality and hysterical personality. Are they 'abnormal'?

Chapter 12

Describe normal psychosexual development. What do you know about homosexuality? How would you proceed when consulted by a man complaining of impotence? Or by a woman complaining of frigidity?
What do you know about morbid jealousy?

Chapter 13

Discuss the concept of psychosomatic reactions, and give examples.
Draw up and study life-charts for patients you have known who had long and complex histories of illness. What can you learn from them?
What is anorexia nervosa?
What is the differential diagnosis of the conditions which may underlie hypochondriasis?

Chapter 14

What factors are involved in the aetiology of alcoholism? What is a typical story of the development of alcoholism? What complications of the condition occur? How is it treated?
Describe the major forms of drug abuse, and how they are treated.

Chapter 15

What is the incidence of mental handicap? Discuss the aetiology, distinguishing between common and rare causes. What services are provided? What are the prospects for prevention?

Chapter 16

How would you proceed when called to the home of a patient who has attempted suicide?

How are emergencies involving aggressive behaviour dealt with?

How are emergencies in acute psychosis treated?

Chapter 17

How have psychiatric services changed in the past thirty years? What are present policies in the provision of facilities for psychiatric patients?

Chapter 18

Discuss the principles of the Mental Health Act (or of the comparable legislation in your country), and describe the main provisions for compulsory admission of those patients who require it. Consider whether you would propose reforms, and if so, why.

How may psychiatric disorders involve patients in breaking the law? What special forms of disposal may be used?

Chapter 19

What is supportive psychotherapy? What is interpretive psychotherapy? What is a therapeutic community?

Discuss: 'Family therapy is not only a new method of treatment but a new way of looking at the problems to be treated'.

Give a general account of the principles of behaviour therapy, and illustrate by specific examples. How different is behaviour therapy from interpretive psychotherapy?

Think about how psychotherapeutic methods have changed since Freud's time. What threads run through the changes? Why may these changes have happened? What do you think about them?

Chapter 20

Describe the main factors bearing upon the development of psychiatric disorders in children.

Compare the clinical approach to a child patient and to an adult.

Describe the prevalence of child psychiatric disorder. What

326 Psychiatry for Students

disorders of eating, sleeping and toilet training are commonly referred for help? How would you help?

Discuss what may lie behind a presenting problem of non-attendance at school.

What is known about childhood psychosis?

Index